30-DAYS HEALTHY GREEN SMOOTHIE PLAN

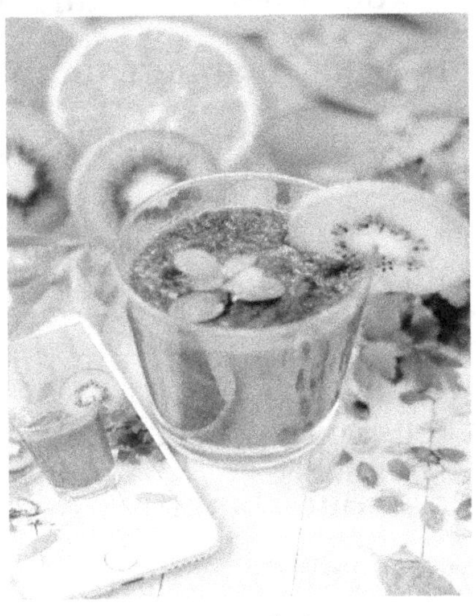

The Best Natural Program For Maximum Weight Loss, Detox & Cleanse

Thelma Pauley

TABLE OF CONTENTS

Introduction

Did you know that the secret to reviving your body, clearing your system, and overcoming weakness may be as easy as making green smoothies your daily habit?

"The 30-Day Green Smoothie Plan" is your passport to detox, cleanse, and weight loss without the fuss. This isn't a crash diet; it's a daily rendezvous with nutrient-packed blends that kickstart your journey to a healthier you. Imagine sipping on easy-to-make green elixirs filled with veggies and fruits – your secret weapon against toxins.

This program offers a whole body and well-being makeover, not just a shift in your regular beverage choice. In a world where severe diets and fast solutions are commonplace in the health space, green smoothies' ease of preparation and nutritional value provide a welcome change of pace.

This plan isn't about deprivation; it's a delicious commitment to feeling lighter, revitalized, and shedding those extra pounds naturally. Get ready for a month-long adventure, where each sip is a step towards a vibrant, energized, and nourished version of yourself. Cheers to a healthier lifestyle!

What Makes Green Smoothies So Good?

Imagine beginning each day with a moment of self-care, a green elixir that sets the tone for renewal, rather than with a rush. Drinking green smoothies is more than simply chasing the latest fashion; it's an investment in your everyday energy and a dedication to your health.

Ease and Availability

The simplicity of green smoothies is their charm. Simple ingredients and easy-to-follow recipes make up this everyday practice that blends in perfectly with your schedule. We'll walk you through the fundamentals to ensure that your trip is both successful and pleasurable.

Food Items Within Reach

Discard the idea that eating well necessitates a complex diet plan and unusual foods. Green smoothies represent our embracing of accessibility. The items you need are probably already waiting in the vegetable department of your neighborhood grocery store, which will serve as your treasure trove. We'll focus on the common and inexpensive, so our approach is not only efficient but also reasonably priced.

Reason For 30-Days

For what reason thirty days? It's a doable period for anyone who is dedicated to enhancing their health, yet it's long enough to see significant results. During this time, we will explore the what, why, and how of green smoothies, learning how they may purify and detoxify our bodies as well as help us overcome the nagging feeling of weakness that keeps us from moving forward.

Examination by Chapter

This journey's chapters are intentionally designed to cover different facets of the 30-day healthy smoothie regimen. We'll progressively provide the groundwork to enable you to include green smoothies into your daily routine in a way that is both sustainable and pleasurable, from understanding the science underlying detoxification to choosing the best ingredients.

Going Beyond the Trend

This is a sustainable way of living, not simply another health trend. As we go into the fundamentals of weight reduction, the significance of exercise, and the craft of customizing your smoothie, the objective isn't only to get you to day 30, but to provide you with skills and habits that last well beyond this period.

Empowerment via Information

We won't overload you with dense ideas and onerous regulations throughout this trip. Rather, the emphasis is on comprehending the underlying concepts of the 30-day nutritious smoothie regimen. You'll discover the benefits of each component for your health, the significance of staying hydrated, and how to customize the flavor combination to suit your palate.

Developing Long-Term Habits

The search for sustainability is essential for improving health. The goal of the chapters on monitoring progress, adjusting lifestyle, and resolving typical problems is to lay a foundation that lasts well beyond the first thirty days. The goal is to enable you to make wise decisions, enjoy the process, and recognize all of your accomplishments, no matter how minor.

Remember that progress, not perfection, is the aim as we set out on our 30-day journey. This flexible guidance, not a set strategy, that will help you figure out what suits you the best. Let's lift our glasses of green smoothies to the upcoming 30 days of rejuvenation, purification, and overcoming our flaws, one drink at a time.

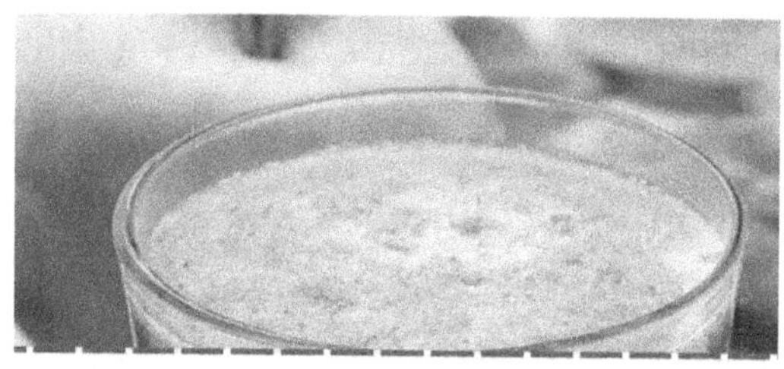

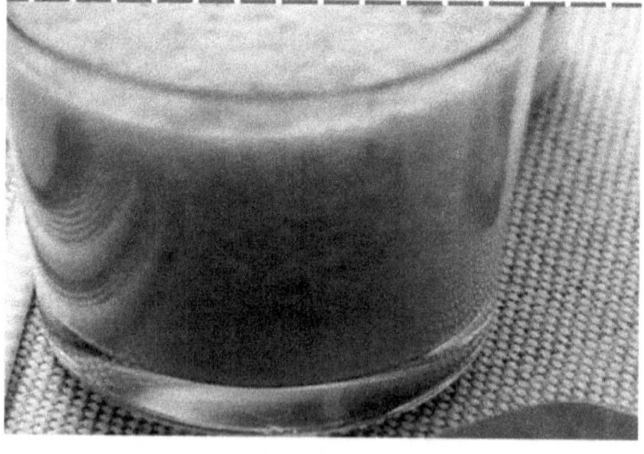

Chapter 1: Understanding Detox, Cleanse, and Weight Loss

Have you ever felt that your body needed a reset button amid life's chaos? Consider it a break for your system, a cleaning, and a more efficient road to improved health. Now, let's break down the basics: Understanding Detox, Cleanse, and Weight Loss:

Detox: It's the body's natural cleanup crew. Consider it like putting out the trash. Detox cleanses your system of stored toxins, allowing your organs to perform more effectively.

Cleanse: This is the maintenance phase, similar to tidying up the mess. Cleanse focuses on your digestive system, enabling a new beginning. It is similar to cleaning your body's pathways.

Weight loss: Think of it as optimizing traffic flow. Shedding extra weight decreases the burden on your body, allowing it to function more smoothly.

It's not only about looking nice; it's about your body performing at its peak. Understanding these factors enables you to set out on a road to becoming a cleaner, leaner, and healthier version of yourself.

Defining Detoxification

Detoxification, often known as detox, is an intriguing and crucial process that occurs naturally in your body and contributes to your general health and well-being. To understand this idea, imagine your body as a bustling city with several systems and functions working constantly to keep everything functioning properly. Consider detox to be the city's waste management system, in charge of cleaning away accumulated garbage and keeping the environment clean and functional.

In its basic form, detoxification is the body's process of eliminating potentially dangerous or unnecessary chemicals. These compounds, often known as toxins, originate from a variety of sources, including the food we consume, the air we breathe, and the stress we feel. Toxins are like uninvited visitors in your city; if left untreated, they may break the serenity.

Now, let's focus on the liver, which plays a key role in the detoxification process. Consider the liver to be the vigilant mayor of the city, monitoring and managing the detoxification process. Toxins are processed to reduce their toxicity before being eliminated from the body by other organs such as the kidneys. This collaboration guarantees that your interior environment remains clean and functioning.

Consider one day in the life of your body. You consume food, breathe in air, and deal with everyday challenges. While these activities are necessary for living, they introduce toxins that must be controlled. This is where detoxification comes in; it is the methodical way your body deals with the effects of daily life.

Detoxing is not about harsh measures or popular cleanses; it is a constant and natural process that promotes your body's optimal functioning. It's similar to regular municipal maintenance, ensuring that the streets are clear and the services are functioning properly. When this process works well, you feel stimulated and your entire health improves.

Now consider what happens when a city's waste management system fails: rubbish accumulates, the air becomes polluted, and the city's vitality suffers. Similarly, if your body's detoxification mechanism fails, pollutants can accumulate, possibly leading to a variety of health problems.

In essence, detoxification protects your interior environment by working relentlessly to preserve balance and harmony. It is not a one-time event, but rather a continual, behind-the-scenes activity that improves your daily well-being. To support this natural process, make toxin-reducing choices, such as eating full, unprocessed foods and properly managing stress.

To summarize, detoxification is your body's internal housekeeping crew, working tirelessly to remove undesirable toxins and maintain a clean, functioning environment. Understanding and respecting this process empowers you to make decisions that promote your body's natural capacity to flourish. So, here's to a well-maintained internal cityscape and a healthier, more energized you!

The Importance of Cleansing in the Wellness Journey

To properly comprehend the necessity of cleaning, consider this intriguing fact: Did you know that your digestive system processes around 10 liters of fluids every day? Consider the impact when this complex system receives the advantages of a well-structured cleansing.

Why Cleaning Matters

Cleansing is more than just a trend; it's an essential part of caring for your health. As your digestive spa, cleaning is critical to preserving your body's equilibrium. Here's why this matters:

1. Nutrient Absorption: A clean digestive tract leads to better nutrition absorption from the diet.

Actionable Step: Eat fiber-rich meals like whole grains and veggies to improve digestive health.

2. Preventing Digestive Buildup: - Consider your digestive tract as a well-traveled highway. Regular cleaning avoids the buildup of undesirable detritus, resulting in easy digestion.

Actionable Step: Drink enough water every day to keep your digestive tract hydrated and encourage effective waste removal.

3. Boosting Energy Levels: - A healthy digestive system leads to improved energy levels. When your body isn't struggling with digestion, you feel more energized.

Actionable Step: Consume probiotic-rich foods such as yogurt to help maintain a healthy balance of gut flora.

4. Supporting Weight control: - Cleansing promotes a balanced approach to weight control, rather than severe methods. It encourages healthy habits and discourages excessive munching.

Actionable Step: Eat smaller, more balanced meals throughout the to help your metabolism.

The Cleansing Process

Understanding the natural cleansing process highlights its significance.

1. Digestive Enzymes: - Enzymes in the digestive tract convert food into nutrients. Cleansing helps these enzymes work more efficiently.

Actionable Step: To help digestion, consume enzyme-rich foods such as papaya or pineapple.

2. Liver and Kidneys:- Your liver and kidneys play a crucial role in detoxification. They digest and remove pollutants, which improves general body function.

 Actionable Step: Reduce your intake of processed foods and alcohol to help your liver.

3. Hydration for Cleansing: - Water aids in eliminating waste and maintaining proper physical processes.

Actionable Step: Drink at least eight glasses of water every day to be well hydrated.

Incorporating Cleansing into Your Routine

Making cleansing a part of your routine doesn't need radical changes.

1. Balanced Nutrition: - Eat a variety of fruits, vegetables, and whole grains for natural cleaning effects.

Actionable Step: Plan colorful, nutrient-dense meals to improve overall wellness.

2. Regular Physical Activity: - Exercise promotes digestion and natural cleaning.

Actionable Step: Choose an activity that you love, such as a daily stroll or a dancing class.

Cleansing isn't a luxury; it's necessary for staying youthful and energetic. Understanding its significance and adding easy procedures into your routine will give you the confidence to enjoy the advantages of a clean body. It's more than simply a chapter in your wellness journey; it's the foundation for a better, more energized existence.

Weight Loss Basics

"Did you know that your body burns calories even while you're still asleep? Let's dive into the fascinating world of weight loss, where knowing the basics is the key to unlocking a healthier, more energized you."

Understanding the Caloric Perplexity

Weight loss isn't just about losing pounds; it's a trip towards well-being. Here's a breakdown of the calorie puzzle:

1. Calories In vs. Calories Out: - Your body weight rests on the balance between calories eaten and calories burned.

Actionable Step: Track your daily food intake to become aware of your calorie usage.

2. Metabolism Matters: - Metabolism affects how many calories your body burns. Muscle mass plays an important part.

Actionable Step: Include strength-training workouts to boost metabolism and keep muscle.

3. Nutrient-Rich Choices: - Opt for nutrient-dense foods; they provide important vitamins and minerals without extra calories.

Actionable Step: Add colorful fruits, veggies, and lean meats to your meals for nutritional benefits.

Portion Control

Understanding portion amounts is important in controlling your weight effectively.

1. Mindful Eating: - Pay attention to what and how much you eat. Mindful eating supports a good connection with food.

Actionable Step: Chew slowly, enjoy each bite, and listen to your body's hunger cues.

2. Plate Composition: - Visualize your plate as a canvas. Fill half with veggies, a quarter protein, and one-quarter with carbs.

Actionable Step: Plate your meals with this visual guide to promote a healthy diet.

Physical Activity and Weight Loss

Exercise isn't just about burning calories; it's a trigger for general well-being.

1. Cardiovascular Exercise: - Activities like walking, running, or riding raise your heart rate and add to calorie burn.

Actionable Step: Aim for at least 150 minutes of moderate-intensity exercise per week.

2. Strength Training: - Building muscle improves metabolism, aiding in long-term weight control.

Actionable Step: Include strength training 2-3 times per week with movements like squats and push-ups.

The Role of Sleep

Quality sleep affects your weight more than you might think.

1. Sleep and Hormones: - Lack of sleep affects hunger hormones, possibly leading to overeating.

Actionable Step: Prioritize 7-9 hours of great sleep each night for general health.

Emotional Eating and Stress Management

Understanding the connection between feelings and

eating is important.

1. Emotional Triggers: - Identify circumstances that lead to emotional eating and develop alternate coping mechanisms.

Actionable Step: Practice deep breathing or invest in a hobby to handle stress.

2. Mindful Stress Reduction: - Chronic worry can add to weight gain. Adopt stress-reducing hobbies like yoga.

Actionable Step: Dedicate a few minutes daily to mindfulness techniques to ease stress.

Hydration and Weight Loss

Water isn't just important for survival; it plays a part in weight management.

1. Hydration and hunger: Drinking water before meals can help reduce hunger.

Actionable Step: Make it a habit to drink a glass of water before each meal.

2. Replacing Sugary Drinks: Opt for water over sugary beverages to lower total calorie intake.

Actionable Step: Choose water or plant teas as your go-to drink

Setting Reasonable Goals

The way to sustainable weight loss involves sensible goals.

1. Gradual Changes: Small, constant changes are more effective than drastic, short-term measures.

Actionable Step: Set realistic goals, such as dropping 1-2 pounds per week.

2. Enjoy Progress: Acknowledge and enjoy milestones, reinforcing good habits.

Actionable Step: Treat yourself with non-food benefits when meeting your goals.

In summary, weight loss isn't a mysterious code but a real journey towards a better lifestyle. By learning the basics and taking small, actionable steps, you empower yourself to make lasting changes for a more energized and vibrant you.

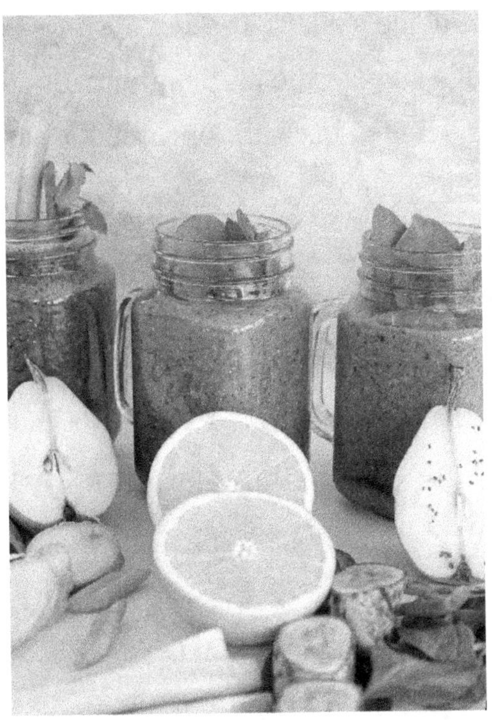

Chapter 2: Benefits of a 30-Day Plan

"Ever heard the saying, 'It takes 21 days to form a habit'? Let's explore the fascinating realm of 30-day plans – a science-backed approach to kickstarting positive change in your life."

The Science Behind 30 Days

Research suggests that committing to a plan for 30 days helps solidify new habits. It's not just a random number; it's a sweet spot for transformation.

Benefits of a 30-Day Plan

1. Establishing Habits

In just 30 days, repetitive actions become ingrained habits. It's like programming your mind and body for positive change.

2. Building Consistency

Consistency is the key to success. A 30-day plan

provides a structured framework, making it easier to stay on track.

3. Measurable Progress

The beauty of 30 days lies in the tangible results you can see. It's like a short journey with milestones that keep you motivated.

4. Breaking the Overwhelm

Long-term goals can be daunting. A 30-day plan breaks them into manageable chunks, reducing overwhelm.

5. Increased Motivation

Short-term goals boost motivation. It's like fuel for your journey, propelling you forward with each passing day.

A 30-day plan is your passport to transformation. It's not just a timeframe; it's a proven strategy to build habits, stay consistent, and witness tangible progress. Embrace the power of 30 days – a simple yet profound approach to kickstarting a positive change in your life.

Establishing Healthy Habits

Ever ponder why it seems so difficult to form or break habits? Let's explore the methods for creating wholesome routines—the tiny yet impactful practices that mold your well-being."

The Science Behind Habits

Comprehending habits is analogous to deciphering your everyday routine. According to research, habits are deeply entrenched actions that are repeatedly carved into the neural pathways of your brain.

The Importance of Healthful Habits

1. Automated Judgments

When you follow healthy habits, making wise judgments comes naturally to you.

2. Steady Progress

Little, regular acts add up over time. Good habits are like building blocks; they all add up to your whole well-being.

3. Energy Conservation

Mental energy is conserved by habits. Once they are in place, they become effective routines that free up mental energy for other work.

4. Emotional Welfare

Emotion is influenced by habits. Making good decisions regularly promotes mental well-being by acting as a little mood booster.

Practical Measures to Form Healthful Routines

1. Identify Trigger Moments

Determine the circumstances that set off your ideal behavior. It is similar to locating the origin of your habit loop.

2. Start Small

Take baby, doable actions to break your habit. It is similar to setting small, manageable goals.

3. Intensity vs Consistency

Regularity triumphs over intensity. Big changes are

always the result of little efforts, like a continuous trickle eroding the rock.

4. Visual Reminders

Set up cues around you to remind you of your habit. It's similar to giving your brain crumbs to follow.

5. Celebrate Milestones

Note accomplishments made along the route. Rewarding little victories is similar to refueling your drive for the next endeavor.

Healthy Habits Examples

1. Daily Stretching Schedule

Begin each day with 5 minutes. It's similar to giving your body a soft embrace when you begin the day.

2. Water Before Meals

A glass of water should be consumed before every meal. It functions similarly to hydrating your body and reducing mindless munching.

3. Thanksgiving Diary

Every day, list three things for which you are

grateful. It's similar to using a few pen strokes to cultivate an optimistic outlook.

Developing healthy behaviors is a steady, doable process rather than an overwhelming endeavor. You may create long-lasting well-being by learning the science underlying habits and putting them into practice with easy, doable actions. Accept the power of little, uplifting habits as your guide to a happier, healthier existence.

Why 30 Days Plan?

"Have you ever wondered why engaging in a 30-day challenge feels like stumbling upon a secret to achieving success? Have you ever pondered why engaging in a 30-day challenge feels like stumbling upon a secret to achieving success? Let's dive into the interesting science behind why 30 days works wonders for transformative change."

The Psychological Power of 30 Days

Research says that it takes approximately 30 days to create a new habit. This timeframe gets into the psychology of habit formation, making it an ideal length for kickstarting positive change.

Key Factors Making 30 Days Effective

1. Repetition Creates Neural Pathways

Doing something regularly for 30 days builds strong neural paths in your brain. It's like creating a well-traveled road, making the action more automatic.

2. Short Enough to Stay Motivated, Long Enough for Impact

A 30-day pledge strikes a balance. It's like starting on a manageable trip – not too short to lose interest, not too long to feel overwhelmed

3. Consistency Builds Energy

Consistency over 30 days creates a sense of energy.

It's like pushing a snowball downhill – small acts build, forming a powerful force for change.

4. Measurable Progress

The 30-day timeframe offers real results. It's like having checkpoints along your trip, allowing you to see and enjoy progress.

Actionable Steps for a Successful 30-Day Challenge

1. Set Clear and Achievable Goals: Define what you want to achieve in 30 days. It's like marking the location on your success map.

2. Break Down Tasks:

Divide your goal into smaller, daily tasks. It's like turning a big job into manageable, bite-sized acts.

3. Daily Tracking:

Keep a log of your daily progress. It's like making a visual record of your trip, letting you stay on track.

4. EnjoyMilestones:

Acknowledge and enjoy successes along the way.

It's like boosting your drive for the next steps.

Examples of Successful 30-Day Challenges

1. Fitness Challenge:

Commit to 30 days of regular workouts. It's like shaping your body one day at a time.

2. Mindfulness Challenge:

Dedicate 10 minutes every day to meditation for a month. It's like making a mental haven over 30 days.

3. Healthy Eating Challenge

Replace processed snacks with fruits and veggies for 30 days. It's like feeding your body with a 30-day restart.

The 30-day magic isn't a myth; it's a scientifically-backed method to making real change. By understanding the psychological aspects, setting clear goals, and adopting consistent actions, you open the potential for transformative success in just 30 days. Embrace the power of this timeframe –

your key to kickstarting positive and lasting changes in your life.

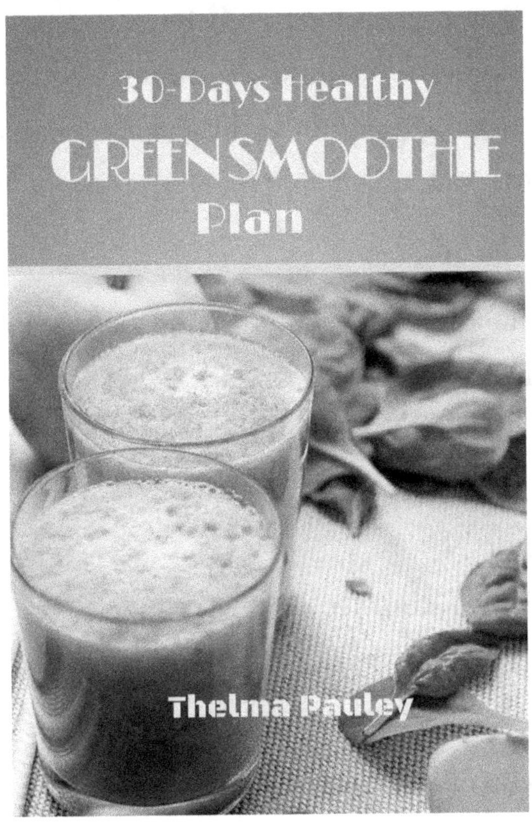

Chapter 3: The Science Behind Green Smoothies

"Have you ever wondered why green smoothies have become a nutritious sensation? Let's look at the science behind these bright mixes, blending statistics, and actionable strategies for a healthy you."

Green smoothies are more than just a craze; they're nutrient-dense. These mixes are high in vitamins and antioxidants, promoting general health.

Why Green Smoothies?

1. Nutrient-Rich Goodness:

Green vegetables, such as spinach and kale, provide critical vitamins, nourishing your body.

2. Digestive Friendliness:

Blending breaks down fiber to improve digestion and nutrition absorption.

3. Hydration Boost:

Green smoothies' high water content promotes

hydration and general wellness.

Making Green Smoothies a Daily Habit

1. Simple Ingredients:

Combine leafy greens, fruits, and liquid to create a tasty and healthy smoothie.

2. Experiment with Flavors:

Tailor your mix to your preferences and make the experience delightful.

3. Maintain consistent green smoothie consumption for long-term health advantages.

In conclusion, green smoothies are more than simply a health craze; they are a scientifically proven technique to provide your body with vital nutrients. With simplicity at their heart, these mixes provide a refreshing and approachable road to optimal nutrition.

Nutritional Components of Green Smoothies

There are many healthy ingredients in green smoothies that work together to make them a great choice for your health. Today we're going to talk about the main health benefits of green smoothies:

1. Leafy Greens: - What They Do

Leafy greens are full of nutrients that your body needs for many processes. They are high in vitamins A, C, and K, as well as folate and iron.

As a step you can take, add spinach, kale, or Swiss chard to your green drinks to make them healthier.

Actionable Step: Vary your vegetables to ensure a broad range of important vitamins and minerals.

Examples of Leafy Greens

Let's delve into the key leafy greens and their unique contributions to a well-balanced diet:

1. Spinach

Nutritional Highlights: Rich in iron, vitamin K,

and folate.

Actionable Tip: Incorporate spinach into salads, smoothies, or sautés for a versatile nutrient boost.

2. Kale

Nutritional Highlights: Packed with vitamins A, C, and K, along with antioxidants.

Actionable Tip: Try kale chips, add them to soups, or blend them into your morning smoothies.

3. Swiss Chard

Nutritional Highlights: A good source of vitamins A, C, and K, as well as magnesium.

Actionable Tip: Sauté Swiss chard with garlic and olive oil for a flavorful side dish.

4. Collard Greens

Nutritional Highlights: High in vitamin K, A, and folate, with anti-inflammatory properties.

Actionable Tip: Include collard greens in wraps or lightly steam for a nutritious side.

5. Arugula

Nutritional Highlights: Rich in vitamins A, C,

and K, and a good source of calcium.

Actionable Tip: Use arugula in salads, sandwiches, or as a pizza topping for a peppery kick.

6. Romaine Lettuce

Nutritional Highlights: A good source of vitamin A, folate, and fiber.

Actionable Tip: Create crisp and refreshing salads with romaine lettuce as the base.

7. Cabbage

Nutritional Highlights: Contains vitamin C, and vitamin K, and is a source of antioxidants.

Actionable Tip: Make coleslaw, add shredded cabbage to stir-fries, or use it in soups.

8. Bok Choy

Nutritional Highlights: Provides vitamins A, C, and K, with a mild, slightly sweet taste.

Actionable Tip: Stir-fry bok choy with garlic and soy sauce for a quick and nutritious side dish.

9. Mustard Greens

Nutritional Highlights: High in vitamins A, C, and K, and rich in antioxidants.

Actionable Tip: Add mustard greens to salads or lightly cook them for a flavorful side.

Incorporating a variety of leafy vegetables into your meals ensures a diverse range of nutrients, supporting overall health and vitality. Experiment with different cooking methods and recipes to make these nutrient-packed greens a delicious and regular part of your diet.

2. Fruits: Role:

Fruits, nature's delicious treasures, offer a wealth of nutrients for your well-being. It adds natural sweetness, fiber, and many vitamins and enzymes.

Step to Take: Add fruits like bananas, berries, or mangoes to make it taste better and give you more nutrients.

Let's delve into the diverse world of fruits and discover how they improve your nutritional intake:

1. Apples

Nutrient Boost: Crunchy and high in fiber, helping digestion.

Versatility: Enjoy as a snack, in salads, or as a natural sweetness in recipes.

2. Bananas

Nutrient Highlights: Packed with potassium, promoting heart health.

Versatile Usage: Perfect for a quick snack, smoothies, or as a natural thickener in baking.

3. Oranges

Nutrient Highlights: Rich in vitamin C for a strong defense system.

Refreshing Delight: Enjoy as a juicy snack or squeeze for fresh zesty drinks.

4. Berries

Nutrient Highlights: Strawberries, blueberries,

and raspberries are antioxidant-rich, helping in cell
defense.

Versatile Usage: Add to cereals, yogurt, or salsa
as a delicious snack.

5. Grapes

Nutrient Highlights: Provide natural sweetness
and contain vitamins.

Snacking Bliss: Enjoy as a handy, refreshing
snack or freeze for a cool treat.

6. Pineapple

Nutrient Goodies: Tropical delight with enzymes
helping digestion.

Culinary Pleasure: Savor as chunks, in fruit
salads, or mixed into drinks.

7. Mango

Nutrient Value: Sweet and filled with vitamins
for skin health.

Versatile Delight: Enjoy sliced, in salsas, or
mixed into delicious mango smoothies.

8. Kiwi

Nutrient Highlights: A small force offering vitamins C and K.

Easy Integration: Peel and enjoy on its own or add to fruit salads for a spicy kick.

9. Peaches

Nutrient Highlights: Juicy and rich in vitamins, supporting general health.

Summer Treat: Enjoy as a solo treat, in sweets, or sliced into salads.

10. Watermelon

Nutrient Hydration: Hydrating and refreshing, great for hot days.

Summer Essential: Delight in slices or blend into a refreshing watermelon drink.

Incorporating these vibrant fruits into your daily diet presents a range of tastes and important nutrients, deliciously supporting your health. From snacks to culinary works, let the natural goodness of fruits improve your nutritional journey.

3. Liquid Base: - Role:

The choice of a liquid base in your culinary endeavors can significantly impact both flavor and nutrition. The liquid part makes sure that everything mixes well and stays moist.

Actionable Step: Use water, coconut water, or almond milk as a base for your green drinks.

Let's explore various liquid bases, their benefits, and how they can elevate your recipes:

1. Water

Clean Hydration: Pure and calorie-free, ideal for maintaining hydration.

2. Coconut Water

Natural Electrolytes: Packed with potassium and electrolytes for hydration.

3. Almond Milk

Nutty Creaminess: Lactose-free and adds a nutty flavor to smoothies or cereals.

4. Greek Yogurt (as a base):

Creamy Texture: Boosts protein content and adds creaminess to smoothies.

5. Orange Juice

Citrus Zest: Provides a burst of vitamin C and a sweet, citrusy flavor.

6. Green Tea (cooled)

Antioxidant Elixir: Adds a subtle, earthy note with the benefits of antioxidants.

7. Pineapple Juice

Tropical Twist: Infuses a tropical flavor, perfect for fruity blends.

8. Milk (Dairy or Plant-Based)

Rich Creaminess: Enhances smoothies with a creamy texture and added nutrients.

9. Aloe Vera Juice

Soothing Elixir: Known for its soothing properties, adds a unique element.

10. Vegetable Broth:

Savory Infusion: For savory smoothies, it provide a different flavor dimension.

Remember to choose your liquid base based on the desired flavor profile and nutritional goals. Whether it's hydration, creaminess, or a hint of flavor, the liquid base can be a transformative element in your culinary creations.

4. Protein Sources: Role:

Green smoothies may be more than simply a cool mix of leafy vegetables; they can also be a whole, high-protein meal or snack. Adding protein sources to your green smoothies boosts their nutritious content while also adding a delicious factor. Protein supports muscle strength and keeps you feeling full. **Actionable Step:** Include sources like Greek yogurt, nut butter, or protein powder for a delicious mix.

Let's look at some high-protein ingredients that can improve the taste of your green smoothie.

1. Yogurt: Greek

Greek yogurt is a smooth and adaptable source of protein that gives your smoothie body a significant amount of high-quality protein. The tart taste of this dairy treat accentuates the freshness of the greens.

2. Protein Powder Made from Plants

Protein powder made from pea, hemp, or brown rice offers a simple and concentrated protein boost for individuals looking for a vegan or plant-based protein choice. It guarantees a balanced nutritional profile without sacrificing flavor.

3. Butter Almond

In addition to adding protein and good fats, almond butter gives your green smoothie a delicious nutty taste. This natural spread provides a pleasing creaminess and improves the flavor.

4. Seeds of Chia

Chia seeds are tiny little powerhouses that are packed full of fiber, protein, and omega-3 fatty acids. They add a hint of crunch and increase the nutritional value of your green smoothie when mixed in.

5. Green Beans

Spinach provides some excellent protein, but it's best recognized for its vitamin and mineral richness. A handful of fresh spinach leaves adds a subtle protein boost to your smoothie while preserving its vivid green hue.

6. Kale

Cruciferous greens like kale are high in vitamins and minerals and are also a good source of protein. Adding kale to your smoothie increases its nutritional richness, which makes it a filling and healthy option.

7. Seeds of Hemp

Being a complete protein source that includes all of the necessary amino acids, hemp seeds stand out. These small seeds are a great addition to green smoothies because they have a nutty taste and provide important protein.

8. Cheese Cottage

Cottage cheese gives your smoothie a smooth smoothness and a powerful protein boost. Its subtle flavor melds well with most fruits and vegetables to provide a filling and healthy combination.

9. Tofu with Silk

A flexible source of protein, silken tofu gives your green smoothie a smooth and creamy texture. It complements fruits and greens effectively, adding a protein boost without drastically changing flavor.

10. Milk (Vegetable or Dairy)

Creaminess and protein are two benefits of adding milk to your green smoothie, whether it's dairy or a plant-based substitute like soy or almond milk. Select the kind of milk that best suits your dietary requirements.

In summary, the secret to a protein-dense green smoothie is the careful blending of various protein sources. Try varying these choices to make your smoothie more to your liking while still making sure it's a healthy, well-balanced part of your diet.

5. Healthy Fats For Smoothies

Green smoothies are a tasty and nourishing way to add healthy fats to your diet, which will enhance the flavor and provide a variety of vital elements. Essential for nutrient intake and general well-being. **Actionable Step:** Add items like avocado, chia seeds, or flaxseeds to add healthy fats.

Let's look at some amazing sources of good fats that can improve the taste of your green smoothie.

The avocado

Avocado is a creamy, nutrient-dense addition to green smoothies and is sometimes referred to as "nature's butter." Rich in monounsaturated fats that are good for the heart, avocados add a mild buttery flavor and velvety texture. They also include vital vitamins, such as potassium and vitamin E, which improve your smoothie's flavor and nutritional value.

2. Seeds of Chia

Chia seeds are not only a great source of protein but also a great source of beneficial omega-3 fatty acids. When combined with liquids, these microscopic seeds expand and take on the consistency of the gel, giving your smoothie a pleasing thickness. Chia seeds include omega-3s that are good for the heart and have anti-inflammatory properties.

3. Seeds of Flax

Ground or as an oil, flaxseeds are a good source of alpha-linolenic acid (ALA), a kind of omega-3 fatty acid. They provide a hint of nutty taste to your smoothie and are good for your heart and general wellness. Furthermore, flaxseeds are a high-fiber food that supports digestive health.

4. Unrefined Coconut Oil

A teaspoon of coconut oil gives your green smoothie a touch of the tropics and adds readily digested lipids called medium-chain triglycerides (MCTs). Because MCTs are well-known for their rapid energy release and their metabolism-boosting properties, coconut oil is a tasty and useful addition.

5. Nuts (Walnuts and Almonds)

Nuts are a great source of healthy fats in addition to being crunchy and tasty. Particularly high in monounsaturated fats and omega-3 fatty acids are almonds and walnuts. By blending these nuts, you may add a wonderful nuttiness and improve the texture of your green smoothie.

6. Seeds of Hemp

Apart from being a good source of protein, hemp seeds are also a good source of omega-3 and omega-6 fatty acids. The subtle nutty flavor of these seeds combines well with the crispness of the greens to create a well-balanced combination of nutrients and flavors.

7. Nut Butter (Peanut and Almond Butter)

Nut butters add protein and healthy fats to your green smoothie, giving it a velvety, decadent texture. For a healthy complement, choose natural types free of hydrogenated oils or added sugars.

8. Olive Oil

Your green smoothie will taste richer with a sprinkle of extra virgin olive oil. Monounsaturated fats found in olive oil are well known for their heart-healthy benefits and delicious texture.

9. Sunflower Seeds

A crunchy and nutrient-rich garnish for green smoothies is sunflower seeds. They are a healthy option since they provide vitamins, minerals, and both mono- and polyunsaturated fats.

10. Seeds From Pumpkins

Pepitas, another name for pumpkin seeds, provide your smoothie with a rich source of healthful lipids and a little crunch. They offer taste and nutrients in the form of omega-3 fatty acids, magnesium, and zinc.

By adding these healthy fat sources to your green smoothies, you can ensure a nutritional composition that is well-rounded while also varying the flavor profile. Try out different combinations to get the ideal mix for your nutritional objectives and taste preferences. Drink a green smoothie to celebrate the health benefits of healthy fats and its vivid, nutrient-rich elixir.

6. Fiber in Green Smoothies

Fiber, often referred to as nature's broom, is an important component that can boost the nutritional content of your green smoothies. Let's explore the importance of fiber and some fiber-rich ads to improve the wholesome goodness of your mix.

Fiber plays a crucial role in supporting gut health, creating a feeling of fullness, and stabilizing blood sugar levels. Incorporating fiber into your green smoothies not only adds to a well-functioning digestive system but also ensures a steady release of energy, making your smoothie a satisfying and healthful choice.

Actionable Step: Keep the fiber level high by including whole fruits and veggies.

Fiber-Rich Additions for Green Smoothies

1. Spinach

Spinach not only adds a bright green hue to your smoothie but is also a great source of fiber. Whether fresh or frozen, spinach easily blends into your concoction, giving both nutritional density and a mild, earthy taste.

2. Kale

Kale, a nutrient powerhouse, provides not only vitamins and minerals but also a large amount of fiber. Blending kale into your green drink improves its fiber content while bringing a slightly peppery note.

3. Chia Seeds

Tiny but strong chia seeds are packed with both soluble and insoluble fiber. When added to your smoothie, they soak liquid and form a gel-like consistency, giving a delicious texture and an extra boost of fiber.

4. Flaxseeds

Flaxseeds, whether ground or in oil form, add a nutty taste and a large dose of fiber to your green smoothie. Additionally, flaxseeds are rich in omega-3 fatty acids, giving a dual benefit.

5. Berries (Blueberries, Strawberries)

Berries bring a burst of sweetness and a substantial amount of fiber to your drink. Blueberries and strawberries, in particular, are rich in antioxidants and add to the total nutritional balance.

6. Avocado

Apart from being a source of healthy fats, avocados are fiber-rich, adding softness and a velvety texture to your green drink. The mix of healthy fats and fiber ensures a delicious and nourishing blend.

7. Apples

Apples, with their natural sweetness and

fiber-packed skin, are excellent adds to green drinks. They give a refreshing taste while contributing to the fiber content and providing a pleasant crunch.

8. Broccoli

Adding a small amount of raw or lightly steamed broccoli to your drink adds a unique taste and a significant fiber boost. Broccoli's flexibility stretches to your green concoction, promoting both taste and nutrition.

9. Cauliflower

Surprisingly flexible, cauliflower can be added to your green drink for a boost of fiber without compromising the taste. It blends well and adds to the general thickness of your blend.

10. Pear

Pears, with their juicy sweetness and fiber-rich flesh, make a delicious addition to green smoothies. They improve the flavor profile while providing a hefty fiber content.

Incorporating these fiber-rich ingredients into your green smoothies not only improves their nutritional value but also adds to a well-balanced and satisfying beverage. Experiment with mixtures to find the right balance of tastes and textures that suit your interests and dietary goals. As you sip on your fiber-rich green drink, relish the healthy benefits that come with each refreshing gulp.

7. Antioxidants in Green Smoothies

Antioxidants are compounds that neutralize harmful free radicals in the body, preventing cellular damage and supporting overall well-being. Including antioxidant-rich foods in your green smoothies enhances their nutritional value and contributes to a vibrant and healthful blend.

Actionable Step: Choose bright ingredients like berries, kiwi, or citrus foods for an antioxidant boost.

Antioxidant-Rich Additions for Green Smoothies

1. Berries (Blueberries, Strawberries, Raspberries)

Berries are brimming with antioxidants, particularly anthocyanins and quercetin. Blueberries, strawberries, and raspberries not only impart a burst of natural sweetness to your smoothie but also offer a colorful array of health-boosting compounds.

2. Spinach

Spinach is not only a fiber powerhouse but also a source of antioxidants, including vitamin C and beta-carotene. The combination of nutrients in spinach supports immune function and contributes to the overall antioxidant capacity of your smoothie.

3. Kale

Kale, a nutrient-dense green, contains antioxidants such as quercetin and kaempferol. Incorporating kale into your green smoothie enhances its antioxidant profile while providing a slightly earthy flavor.

4. Green Tea (cooled)

Green tea is rich in catechins, powerful antioxidants with various health benefits. Adding cooled green tea to your smoothie imparts a subtle earthy note while infusing your blend with antioxidant goodness.

5. Cinnamon

Beyond its warm and comforting flavor, cinnamon boasts antioxidant properties. A sprinkle of cinnamon in your green smoothie not only enhances its taste but also contributes to the overall antioxidant content.

6. Dark Chocolate (Cocoa)

Unsweetened dark chocolate or cocoa powder is a delightful addition to your green smoothie, offering flavonoids with antioxidant activity. This indulgent touch elevates both the flavor and nutritional profile of your blend.

7. Pomegranate Seeds

Pomegranate seeds are a rich source of antioxidants, particularly punicalagin and anthocyanins. These ruby-red gems add a burst of sweetness and a unique texture to your green smoothie while boosting its antioxidant content.

8. Ginger

Ginger contains potent antioxidants, including gingerol. Adding a small piece of fresh ginger to your smoothie not only provides a zesty kick but also contributes to the overall antioxidant capacity.

9. Turmeric

Curcumin, the active compound in turmeric, is known for its antioxidant and anti-inflammatory properties. Including a pinch of turmeric in your green smoothie not only adds a warm, earthy flavor but also enhances its health-promoting qualities.

10. Acai Berry Puree

Acai berries are well known for their antioxidant content, particularly anthocyanins. Incorporating acai berry puree into your green smoothie introduces a delightful berry flavor while amplifying its antioxidant potential.

By incorporating these antioxidant-rich ingredients into your green smoothies, you not only enhance their flavor but also create a nutritional powerhouse. Experiment with combinations to find the perfect blend that suits your taste preferences and harnesses the vibrant benefits of antioxidants with every sip.

8. Vitamins and Minerals

Green smoothies serve as a vibrant canvas for an array of important vitamins and minerals, adding to general health and well-being. Let's explore the nutrient-rich adds that can turn your green smoothie into a powerhouse of vitamins and minerals.

Vitamins and minerals are important micronutrients that play varied roles in supporting bodily processes. Incorporating a range of nutrient-dense vegetables in your green smoothies ensures a well-rounded supply of these important elements, promoting optimal health.

Vitamin and Mineral-Rich Additions for Green Smoothies

1. Spinach

Spinach is a nutritional wonder, offering a rich source of vitamins A, C, and K, and minerals such as iron and magnesium. Adding spinach to your green smoothie adds to its bright green color and improves its nutritional profile.

2. Kale

Kale, a leafy green wonder, is filled with vitamins A, C, and K, as well as minerals like calcium and manganese. Including kale in your green drink not only adds a robust taste but also boosts its vitamin and mineral content.

3. Banana

Bananas are not only a natural sweetener for your drink but also a source of vitamins B6 and C, potassium, and manganese. Their creamy texture compliments the general consistency of your blend.

4. Avocado

Avocado, besides giving healthy fats, adds vitamins E, K, C, and B-complex, along with minerals like potassium and folate. Avocado improves the creaminess of your smoothie while adding a subtle, buttery flavor.

5. Berries (Blueberries, Strawberries)

Berries bring a burst of taste and a wealth of vitamins and antioxidants to your green drink. Blueberries and strawberries, in particular, offer vitamins C and K, as well as manganese.

6. Oranges (Drink or Parts)

Oranges, whether in drink form or as segments, fill your smoothie with vitamin C, potassium, and folate. The citrusy brightness improves the total taste and nutritional value.

7. Mango

Mango adds tropical sweetness to your green drink while adding vitamins A, C, and E, along with minerals like potassium and magnesium. Its vibrant taste matches the freshness of veggies.

8. Greek Yogurt

Greek yogurt not only gives protein but also provides calcium, vitamin B12, and probiotics. The creamy texture and tangy taste make it a flexible addition to your green smoothie.

9. Pineapple

Pineapple brings a delicious tropical twist to your drink, along with vitamins C and manganese. Its natural sweetness balances the taste while adding to the nutrient content.

10. Kiwi

Kiwi is a vitamin C powerhouse and also offers vitamins K and E. Adding kiwi to your green smoothie brings a unique tartness and a burst of important nutrients.

By adding these vitamin and mineral-rich items to your green smoothies, you create a delicious and nutrient-dense elixir. Experiment with different mixtures to find the perfect blend that suits your taste preferences and ensures a wide array of vitamins and minerals with every sip.

How Green Smoothies Aid Detox and Weight Loss

In the drive for a healthy lifestyle, the intersection of detoxification and weight loss has become a focus point for many people. Green smoothies, with their bright colors and nutrient-packed ingredients, emerge as a powerhouse in supporting both detox and weight loss efforts. Let's dive into the complex dance between green smoothies, detoxification, and losing those extra pounds.

Detoxification Simplified

Detoxification, often referred to as detox, is the normal process by which the body removes or neutralizes poisons. These toxins can come from various sources, including processed foods, environmental pollutants, and everyday stresses. The organs involved in detoxification, such as the liver, kidneys, and digestive system, work constantly to clear out and remove these unwanted substances.

Green Smoothies as Detox Elixirs

Green smoothies – a mixture of fresh, leafy veggies, fruits, and nutrient-rich additions. The chlorophyll in leafy veggies, the fiber in fruits, and the antioxidants in different ingredients all play vital parts in supporting the body's natural detox processes.

1. Chlorophyll Boost

Leafy veggies like spinach and kale are rich in chlorophyll, the green pigment responsible for photosynthesis. Chlorophyll has been studied for its ability to aid detoxification by binding to toxins and helping their removal from the body.

2. Fiber Magic

The fiber content in green smoothies, courtesy of ingredients like fruits and veggies, works as a natural broom for your digestive system. Fiber supports regular bowel movements, avoiding the buildup of waste and enabling the efficient removal of toxins.

3. Hydration Hurdle

Green smoothies, often built on a liquid basis, add to hydration. Proper hydration is important for kidney health, one of the key players in cleansing. Fluids help move waste products for elimination, keeping your detox routes well-lubricated.

4. Antioxidant Arsenal

Berries, citrus fruits, and other antioxidant-rich add to green smoothies provide a strong defense against oxidative stress. Oxidative stress happens when there's an imbalance between free radicals and antioxidants in the body, and it's involved in different health problems. By arming your body with antioxidants, green smoothies help eliminate free radicals and support general well-being.

Harmonizing Nutrition and Caloric Control

Weight loss is a complicated interplay of caloric intake, metabolism, and living choices. While it's important to create a caloric deficit (burning more calories than you consume), the quality of those calories counts too. Green smoothies step onto the weight loss stage by giving a nutrient-dense, low-calorie choice that can be a valuable addition to a balanced diet.

Green Smoothies as Weight Loss Allies

1. Nutrient Density

Green drinks pack a healthy punch with vitamins, minerals, and phytonutrients, all while keeping calorie counts in check. This nutrient density is important for giving necessary elements without the extra calories often found in processed or high-fat foods.

2. Fiber for Satiety

The fiber level in green smoothies promotes a feeling of fullness and satisfaction. This can be instrumental in preventing unnecessary snacking or overeating, adding to better portion control and obedience to a calorie-controlled diet.

3. Balanced Nutrition

A well-constructed green smoothie can include a mix of macronutrients – carbs, protein, and healthy fats. This balance is beneficial to sustained energy levels, helping you stay busy and keep a more regular caloric burn throughout the day.

4. Hydration and Metabolism

Proper hydration is important for general health, and green smoothies add to your fluid diet. Additionally, water helps metabolic processes, including the breakdown of stored fat. A well-hydrated body is more efficient at utilizing energy, possibly helping in weight loss.

5. Natural Detox Support

As mentioned earlier, the detoxifying qualities of green smoothies indirectly support weight loss. A body free of excess toxins may work more optimally, possibly improving metabolism and general health.

Practical Tips for Detox and Weight Loss

1. Diverse Greens: Experiment with a range of leafy greens like spinach, kale, and Swiss chard to vary your vitamin intake.

2. Colorful Additions: Incorporate a variety of colorful fruits and veggies to ensure a broad range of vitamins, minerals, and antioxidants.

3. Hydration Emphasis: Use water, coconut water, or unsweetened almond milk as your liquid base to emphasize hydration without extra sugars.

4. Mindful Ingredients: Be aware of ingredient choices to keep a balance between nutrition richness and caloric content.

5. Gradual Integration: If new to green drinks, start gradually to allow your taste buds to change. You can begin with milder greens and gradually raise the strength.

6. Consistency is Key: Consider adding green drinks into your routine regularly. Whether as a meal replacement or a snack, regular drinking can add to continued detoxification and weight loss efforts.

Green smoothies appear as flexible instruments in the music of health, playing harmonious tunes that support both detoxification and weight loss. Their nutrient-rich composition, hydrating qualities, and potential for caloric control make them useful adds to a health-conscious lifestyle. As you sip on your bright green elixir, relish in the knowledge that each gulp adds not only to your taste buds but also

to the complex dance of detoxification and weight
loss within your body.

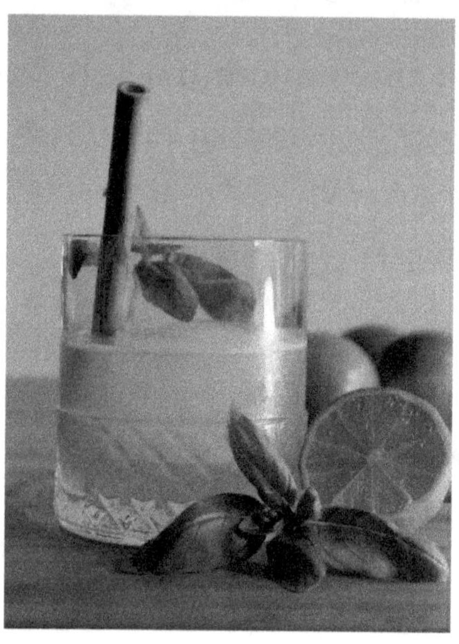

Chapter 4: Types of Green Smoothies

Green smoothies come in various types, mixing leafy veggies with fruits and liquids. Classic ones feature spinach or kale with banana and water. Detox mixes include parsley, cucumber, and lemon for a delicious twist. Experiment with items to find your favorite nutritious mix!

Power-packed green drinks often include vegetables like kale, spinach, or chard, paired with fruits like berries, pineapple, and mango. Adding a liquid base like water, coconut water, or almond milk makes a tasty and healthy drink that's easy to whip up for a quick nutrient boost.

For an energy kick, try adding items like chia seeds, flaxseeds, or a scoop of protein powder. These nutrient-dense blends not only offer a burst of vitamins but also make a delicious and handy way to add greens to your daily routine. Experimenting with amounts lets you tailor your smoothie to personal taste and health goals.

Fruit-Based Smoothies

Fruit-based smoothies are like the superheroes of drinks – a mix of fruits, leafy greens, and fluids. Imagine a superhero team where spinach, banana, and water join forces for the greater good of your well-being.

So, why should you care about these liquid concoctions? It's simple – they're a tasty way to get lots of nutrients. Picture this: spinach and fruits teaming up in your blender to make a power-packed drink that's not only delicious but also a vitamin powerhouse.

Types of Fruit-Based Smoothies

1. Leafy Greens Base

Let's start with the basics – the Leafy Greens Base. It's like the OG (Original Green) drink. Spinach or kale teams up with banana and water, making a smooth blend that's an easy starting point into the world of green goodness.

2. Detox Blend

Do you feel like you need a reset button? Enter the Detox Blend. This one's like a refreshing shower for your insides. Imagine parsley, cucumber, and lemon working together to give your body a gentle cleaning.

3. Berries and Greens

Now, imagine a Berry Blast. Berries and Greens drink brings together the goodness of kale or spinach with the sweetness of blueberries or strawberries. It's like a sweet party in your mouth.

4. Tropical Fusion

If you're thinking of a tropical trip, the Tropical Fusion smoothie is your ticket. Spinach or kale takes a trip with pineapple and mango, making a vacation-like vibe in your blender.

5. Protein Boost

Need a little extra kick? The Protein Boost drink is here to save the day. Add chia seeds, flaxseeds, or protein powder, and suddenly your smoothie is not just a drink – it's a fuel station for your day.

6. Citrus Splash Smoothie

A zesty mix of oranges, grapefruits, and a handful of spinach, makes a tangy and refreshing concoction that wakes up your taste buds.

7. Mango Madness Smoothie

Dive into tropical happiness with a mix of ripe mango, banana, and coconut water, transporting you to an exotic heaven with every sip.

8. Berry Citrus Burst

A bright blend of strawberries, blueberries, and a splash of orange juice, marrying the sweetness of berries with the citrusy kick for a flavorful explosion.

9. Pineapple Passion Smoothie

Savor the tropical goodness of pineapple mixed with passion fruit and a hint of mint, creating a breezy and delightful blend reminiscent of a beachside escape.

10. Apple Pie Delight

Experience the taste of fall with a mix of apples, cinnamon, and a touch of oats, mimicking the cozy flavors of a classic apple pie in liquid form.

11. Tropical Green Tea Infusion

Elevate your smoothie game by mixing green tea with pineapple, kiwi, and a handful of spinach, making a bright and antioxidant-rich beverage.

12. Peachy Keen Creamsicle

A creamy fusion of peaches, vanilla yogurt, and a splash of orange juice, gives a peachy creamsicle treat that feels like pie in a glass.

13. Cherry Almond Bliss

Cherries meet almond milk and a scoop of almond

butter, making a luscious and nutty smoothie that's both indulgent and healthy.

14. Watermelon Mint Refresher

Stay hydrated with a watermelon-based smoothie, mixed with fresh mint leaves, giving a cooling and hydrating treat great for hot days.

14. Dragon Fruit Elegance

Step into the exotic with dragon fruit, mixed berries, and coconut water, making a visually stunning and delicious drink packed with antioxidants.

In a word, fruit-based smoothies are your ticket to a tasty and healthy journey. From the basic Leafy Greens to the tropical adventure of Tropical Fusion, each sip is a step towards a healthy you.

So, grab that mixer, throw in some fruits and veggies, and let the fruity music begin – a harmonious blend of health and happiness, one smoothie at a time. Cheers to the easy joy of sipping your way to health!

Vegetable-Based Smoothies

"Forget everything you thought you knew about veggies – we're about to blend them into a whole new level of goodness. Welcome to the world of Vegetable-Based Smoothies, where nutrition meets creativity in a mixer!"

Vegetable-based drinks may sound odd, but trust us, they're a game-changer for your health. Imagine sipping on a beverage that not only tastes surprisingly good but also feeds your body with the goodness of veggies. Let's dive into this vibrant world where broccoli, carrots, and kale change into liquid vitality.

What's the deal with vegetable-based smoothies? Think of it as a special drink where veggies take center stage alongside fruits and liquids. It's a delightful way to sneak in those nutrient-packed greens, making your daily dose of veggies a sip away.

Types of Vegetable-Based Smoothies

1. Verdant Veggie Oasis Smoothie

The ultimate green treat features spinach, cucumber, and celery, making a garden-fresh smoothie that's both hydrating and healthy.

2. Carrot Cake Fusion Smoothie

Sip on the essence of carrot cake with this blended concoction of carrots, cinnamon, and almond milk – a wholesome and flavorful twist in liquid form.

3. Tomato Basil Smoothies

Tomatoes meet fresh basil and a hint of balsamic vinegar, making a savory and filling smoothie that's a change from the sweet standard.

4. Broccoli Pineapple Fusion

Break the mold with a surprising duo – broccoli and pineapple – joining for a sweet and savory blend that's as healthy as it is tasty.

5. Sweet Potato Spice Bliss Smoothie

Indulge in the warmth of sweet potatoes, nutmeg, and coconut milk with this delightful and spiced smoothie – a comforting treat that's both flavorful and nutritious.

6. Cucumber Mint Refresher

Embrace crisp refreshment with cucumber, mint, and a squeeze of lime, making a hydrating and revitalizing drink great for a sunny day.

7. Avocado Berry Boost

Avocado joins forces with mixed berries and a touch of honey, resulting in a creamy and antioxidant-rich smoothie that's both filling and healthy.

8. Spinach Mango Tango

Spinach pairs up with the sweetness of mango and a hint of ginger, dancing together in a tropical-flavored blend that's as healthy as it is delicious.

9. Bell Pepper Citrus Splash

Red or yellow bell peppers meet citrus fruits like oranges and a touch of honey, making a vitamin C-packed smoothie with a delicious tang.

10. Zucchini Chocolate Indulgence

Yes, you read it right – zucchini and chocolate! Blend zucchini with cocoa powder and a banana for a guilt-free, sweet treat that sneaks in extra veggies.

11. Kale Pineapple Paradise

Immerse yourself in the lush tastes of kale and pineapple, creating a tropical paradise in a glass that's both energizing and packed with nutrients.

12. Cauliflower Blueberry Bliss

Embrace the unexpected with broccoli mixed with blueberries and a splash of almond milk, resulting in a creamy and antioxidant-rich smoothie.

13. Asparagus Apple Orchard

Step into a refreshing garden of flavors by mixing asparagus with apples and a hint of mint, creating a unique smoothie with a crisp twist.

14. Beet Berry Burst

Unleash the bright colors and benefits of beets in a berry-infused smoothie, where the earthiness of beets compliments the sweetness of mixed berries.

15. Radish Lemonade Refresher

Elevate your taste buds with the zingy mix of radishes, lemon, and a touch of honey, creating a revitalizing and tangy drink reminiscent of homemade lemonade.

From the green goodness of spinach to the surprising joy of zucchini and chocolate, vegetable-based smoothies rethink the way we eat veggies. So, grab your blender and start on a flavorful trip where vegetables take on a whole new, sip-worthy identity. Cheers to vegetable-based vibrance and a better, tastier you!

Protein-Enhanced Smoothies

Protein-enhanced smoothies are the stars of the blending world. Imagine filling your body with not just taste but also the power of protein. This is not your normal smoothie; it's a delicious elixir meant to support your muscles and keep you going strong.

Why the protein obsession? Picture this: proteins are the building blocks for muscles, and a protein-enhanced drink is like a construction site for your body. It's a tasty way to ensure you're not just sipping but also supporting your muscles.

Types of Protein-Enhanced Smoothies

1. Basic Banana Protein Boost

Start with a basic – banana, protein powder, and almond milk. This drink not only tastes like a treat but also gives your muscles the protein kick they need.

2. Berry Protein Punch

Berries join the protein party! Blend mixed berries with Greek yogurt and a scoop of protein powder for a sweet burst that's also a protein powerhouse.

3. Peanut Butter Chocolate Delight

Indulge without worry. Combine peanut butter, chocolate protein powder, and a banana for a creamy and decadent shake that's also a protein-packed wonder.

4. Green Protein Revival

Revitalize with greens! Spinach, banana, and a scoop of protein powder make a green drink that's not just refreshing but also a protein-enhanced energy booster.

5. Coffee Protein Buzz

Wake up and power up! Brewed coffee, protein powder, and a splash of almond milk make a coffee-flavored protein smoothie, giving you a morning buzz with extra benefits.

6. Tropical Protein Paradise

Escape to the tropics with a mix of pineapple, coconut milk, and vanilla protein powder, making a refreshing and protein-packed smoothie that feels like a beach trip.

7. Almond Joy Infusion

Indulge in the tastes of an Almond Joy candy bar by blending almond butter, coconut bits, chocolate protein powder, and almond milk for a delicious and protein-rich treat.

8. Chia Seed Protein Booster

Elevate your drink with chia seeds! Combine them with fruit, vanilla protein powder, and almond milk for a textured and protein-enhanced treat.

9. Mango Turmeric Protein Elixir

Embrace the anti-inflammatory benefits by mixing mango, turmeric, a bit of ginger, and protein powder, making a tropical elixir that supports your muscles and general well-being.

10. Blueberry Oatmeal Powerhouse

Fuel up with oats! Blend blueberries, oats, and a scoop of protein powder with milk for a filling and protein-enhanced smoothie that's perfect for a satisfying breakfast or post-workout refuel.

11. Spinach Avocado Protein Boost

Go green and creamy! Combine spinach, avocado, banana, and protein powder for a nutrient-packed and protein-rich smoothie that's as healthy as it is delicious.

12. Strawberry Kiwi Protein Refresher

Quench your thirst with a mix of strawberries, kiwi, and protein powder, making a fruity and hydrating smoothie that packs a protein punch.

13. Pumpkin Spice Protein Indulgence

Embrace the tastes of fall! Blend pumpkin puree, cinnamon, vanilla protein powder, and almond milk for a holiday joy that's both comforting and protein-rich.

14. Peach Almond Protein Smoothies

Enjoy the balance of peaches and nuts! Blend fresh peaches, almond butter, and protein powder for a shake that's not only delicious but also a protein-packed treat.

15. Raspberry Mint Protein Smoothies

Refresh and refuel with a mix of raspberries, fresh mint leaves, and protein powder, making a vibrant and protein-enhanced smoothie that tingles the taste buds.

From classic banana to the coffee-infused buzz, protein-enhanced smoothies rethink the art of mixing. So, whether you're a fitness lover or just love a good-tasting, muscle-loving drink, dive into the world of protein-powered bliss. Sip, enjoy, and improve – here's to a tastier and healthier you!

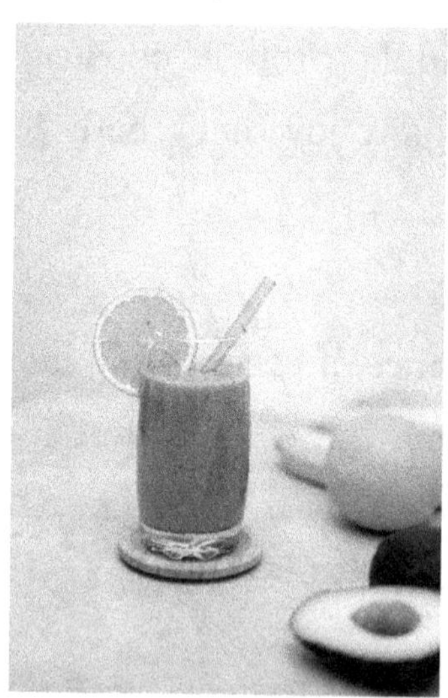

Chapter 5: The Right Blend for the Blend

To prepare a delicious green smoothie, picture yourself as assembling a wonderful team. First, choose leafy greens; they are superfood superheroes. Add some fruits for extra nutrition and sweetness. Like a captain of the squad, the liquid base maintains order. Remember that protein provides power, and healthy fats provide texture. In addition to antioxidants serving as your defense, fiber aids with digestion. Lastly, the scene is set with vitamins and minerals. As the coach, picture yourself combining these components to form a winning squad for your well-being.

Put another way, the key to making the ideal green smoothie is selecting the proper ratio of fruits and vegetables. For a nutritious green basis, start with a handful of raw spinach or kale. To make it creamy and sweet, add a banana. Add some berries for an antioxidant and taste boost. A slice of pineapple can work if you want it tart. Remember to add a little liquid, such as orange juice, coconut water, or even just water. Mix everything until it's smooth and served! Try out many combinations to discover the one that satisfies your palate and is high in nutrients.

Choosing Your Green Smoothie Ally

Making the ideal green smoothie is more than just experimenting with tastes; it's a deliberate choice to live a more energetic, healthier existence. Choosing your green smoothie pals is an essential responsibility at the center of this lush quest. These friends, which include fruits, leafy greens, healthy fats, and vital nutrients, each have a unique function in enhancing the nutritional value and flavor of your smoothie.

We will explore the diverse realm of green smoothie pals in this chapter, identifying the special qualities that each adds to the blender's canvas. Learn about the subtleties of selecting the best leafy greens, the function of healthy fats, the delicious symphony created by fruits, and the essential minerals and vitamins that enhance health advantages. Come along for a delicious, simple journey as we walk you through the process of choosing the ideal companions for your green smoothie, bringing every mouthful a step closer to health and deliciousness.

In this guide, we'll look at your green smoothie allies: the simple, delightful components that will make your drink not only delicious but also beneficial to your health. So, let's have a look at how to choose your ideal green smoothie buddies in an easy-to-understand and enjoyable manner!

The first step in creating a delicious green smoothie is selecting the appropriate leafy greens. They're like your trusty aides on this green trip. In this extensive tutorial, we'll look at how to pick the best green smoothie ingredients, including spinach, kale, and Swiss chard. And the greatest part? We'll accomplish it without utilizing complex vocabulary or clever comparisons. It's all about keeping things simple and easy to grasp.

Leafy Green As a Smoothie Allies

Leafy greens are the hidden heroes of the green smoothie landscape, providing a wealth of nutrients that promote general health. Spinach, kale, and Swiss chard are among the best contenders to be your smoothie buddies. Each of these greens offers a distinct flavor to the table, catering to a variety of taste preferences and nutritional requirements.

1. Spinach: Mild-Mannered Contender

Spinach is the Clark Kent of leafy greens, modest but full of nutritious strength. Its moderate flavor profile makes it an ideal choice for people looking to incorporate green food into their diet without overwhelming their taste receptors. Spinach contains a high concentration of important vitamins, including A and C. Vitamin A promotes eye health, but vitamin C strengthens the immune system.

Furthermore, spinach contains a significant amount of iron, which is essential for keeping healthy blood and avoiding anemia. Its flexibility goes beyond smoothies, making it an ideal choice for a variety of culinary applications. Using fresh, colorful spinach leaves maximizes the nutritional value of your green elixir.

2. Kale: The Robust Champion

Kale enters the smoothie scene with a strong and earthy presence. This powerful green leafy vegetable is well-known for its nutritional contents, giving it the title of "green powerhouse." Kale packs a powerful health punch, thanks to its antioxidants, fiber, and a variety of vitamins such as K, A, and C.

Kale's fiber content supports digestive health and satiety, making it a good option for people looking to maintain a healthy weight. Kale's antioxidants promote general health by countering oxidative stress in the body. While kale's flavor may be more intense, its nutritional advantages make it an excellent companion in the goal of a nutrient-dense green smoothie.

3. Swiss Chard: The Colorful Surprise

Swiss chard emerges as the underdog, enticing smoothie fans with its vivid stems and soft leaves. This versatile green has a milder flavor than kale, making it a more inviting option for those new to the world of green smoothies. The visual appeal of Swiss chard provides a bright flare to your beverage, making it both aesthetically pleasant and nutritional.

Swiss chard has a wide nutritional profile, which includes vitamins A, K, and C, as well as minerals like magnesium and potassium. The combination of these nutrients promotes a variety of body processes, including bone health (thanks to vitamin K) and electrolyte balance (courtesy of magnesium and potassium). Including Swiss chard in your green smoothie recipes provides a delicious combination of taste and nutrients.

Freshness is Key: The Importance of Bright Greens

Regardless of your chosen green ally, the key to a great green smoothie is to use fresh ingredients. Choose bright, fresh leaves with no evidence of wilting or browning. Fresh greens not only improve the flavor of your smoothie, but they also ensure that you receive the most nutritional value out of your chosen ingredients.

Preparation: Converting Greens to Liquid Gold

Once you've chosen your leafy greens, preparing them for blending is a simple task. Wash the leaves well to eliminate any dirt and contaminants. Removing tough stems is suggested, especially for kale and Swiss chard, as it produces a nicer texture in the finished product.

Toss your greens into the blender and watch as they change into a nutrient-rich miracle. Experimentation is essential for finding the ideal mix that matches your taste buds and nutritional goals. Consider blending various greens to create a symphony of flavors and optimize the variety of nutrients they provide.

Finally, the world of green smoothies offers a plethora of options for both your taste buds and your health. Whether you like the subtle appeal of spinach, the powerful character of kale, or the brilliant variety of Swiss chard, each green ally adds its nutritious value to your cup. Freshness is essential, and a little experimenting allows you to customize your smoothie to your tastes.

So, think of your blender as an artist's canvas where you mix lots of colorful greens. Then, sip your way to feeling healthier and more lively! The path to a nutrient-rich, tasty green smoothie is not only simple but also a rewarding discovery of healthful components that promote your well-being.

Fruits As Your Smoothie Allies

Green smoothies are built based on leafy greens, with fruits adding sweetness and crucial minerals. Exploring this delicious combination of tastes and goodness doesn't take any culinary knowledge; it's simply a journey through the lively world of fruits and learning how each contributes to the creation of a pleasant and healthy drink.

Bananas: The Creamy Sweethearts

Bananas, with their natural sweetness and creamy texture, are the perfect addition to any green smoothie. They not only offer a delicious flavor but also improve the overall consistency of your mix, making it velvety and enjoyable. Beyond their flavor, bananas are high in potassium, a mineral that promotes heart health and helps the body maintain optimal water levels.

When picking bananas for your smoothie, use ripe bananas with yellow skins. This offers the perfect sweetness and a smoother mixing experience.

Simply peel, slice, and mix them for a pleasantly creamy addition to your green smoothie.

Berries: Colorful and Healthy Bites

Berries, such as strawberries and blueberries, provide a splash of color to your green smoothie while also providing several health advantages. These small nibbles are not only delightful, but they are also high in vitamins, notably vitamin C, which is known to improve the immune system. Berries offer a delicious flavor to your mix while also providing antioxidants to prevent oxidative stress in the body.

Experimenting with different berry combinations allows you to customize the flavor of your smoothie. Berries, whether fresh or frozen, are a flexible and easily available addition to your beverage, adding flavor as well as nutritional content.

Mango: The Tropical Treat

Mangoes provide a tropical twist to your green smoothie, infusing it with a bright, exotic flavor. Aside from their excellent taste, mangoes are high in vitamins A and C. Vitamin A improves eyesight, whilst vitamin C boosts immunological function and stimulates collagen creation for good skin.

To make a mango smoothie, peel and dice the fruit, discarding the huge pit. Mango's natural sweetness and tropical flair give your green smoothie a lovely touch, making it feel like a refreshing retreat.

Pineapple: The Refreshing Addition

Pineapple, with its tart and refreshing flavor, is an excellent addition to any green smoothie. Loaded with vitamin C and manganese, pineapple improves immunological function and adds to bone health. Its distinct flavor provides a refreshing sensation, making your smoothie more delightful, particularly on warm days.

When adding pineapple to your mix, you can use fresh or frozen pieces. For a smooth and tasty product, ensure that the pineapple is peeled and cored before blending.

Apples and Pears: Crispy Goodness

Apples and pears give your green smoothie a crunchy texture and natural sweetness, making it a nutritious and enjoyable beverage. These fruits are high in dietary fiber, which promotes digestive health and provides a consistent flow of energy.

Preparing apples and pears for a smoothie is simple. Core and slice into manageable pieces, making sure they combine well with the other ingredients. The mix of their sharpness and natural sweetness improves the overall flavor of your green beverage.

Creating Your Fruit Mix

The beauty of green smoothies is the ability to experiment and adapt the combination to your tastes. Whether you choose a berry blend, a tropical infusion, or the classic combo of apples and pears, the options are endless and delicious. Allow your taste sensations to lead you as you experiment with different fruit combinations, seeking the ideal mix of sweetness and nutrients.

Tips for Success When Adding Fruits to Your Smoothie

1, Freshness Matters

Choose ripe, fresh fruits for the best flavor and nutritional value. If you use frozen fruits, be sure they are devoid of chemicals and preservatives.

2. Preparation

Peel, slice, and prep your fruits to ensure they combine easily in your smoothie. Removing cores, pits, and inedible pieces allows for a more delightful drinking experience.

3. Portion Control

While fruits provide natural sugars and critical nutrients, they must be consumed in moderation. Consider your smoothie's total nutritional makeup when deciding on serving sizes.

Finally, fruits are active companions in your green smoothie adventure, providing sweetness, texture, and a variety of critical nutrients. Bananas add smoothness, berries add color and health, mangoes provide a tropical delight, pineapples add freshness, and apples or pears add crunchy deliciousness.

So, let your blender turn this fruity mixture into a delectable elixir, and drink your way to a healthier, happier you. Cheers to the simple joy of greens and fruits in your green smoothie voyage, where each drink is a wonderful step toward better health!

Liquid Base: An Essential Green Smoothie Allies

As we continue our journey into the art of creating the ultimate green smoothie, let's focus on the often-overlooked hero: liquid base. The liquid base, like the conductor of an orchestra, sets the tempo for your smoothie symphony, resulting in a harmonic balance of flavors and a fluid texture. In this article, we'll look at the most important factors in choosing the best liquid basis for your verdant concoction.

1. Water: The Pure Hydration Conductor

Water, the most basic and pure of ingredients, serves as the underlying conductor for your green smoothie. Water provides hydration without changing the flavor profile, allowing the natural essence of leafy greens and fruits to show through. It's a wonderful choice for people who want a clean, sharp canvas for their smoothie creation.

Ensure the quality of your water by selecting filtered or purified choices. Add water gradually while mixing until you reach the appropriate consistency, allowing you to adjust the texture of your green elixir.

2. Coconut Water: The Tropical Serenade

Coconut water is an excellent beverage companion for adding a bit of tropical flare. Coconut water, which is high in electrolytes and has a mild sweetness, pairs well with the earthy tones of greens and provides a refreshing twist to your smoothie symphony. It's especially well-suited for individuals who enjoy a bit of tropical pleasure with each drink.

To keep your green smoothie's healthy theme, use pure, unsweetened coconut water. Coconut water's electrolyte content helps to keep you hydrated, making it a good choice for individuals who lead an active lifestyle.

3. Nut Milk (Almond, Cashew, etc.): A Creamy Crescendo

Nut milk, such as almond or cashew adds a velvety finish to your green smoothie. These dairy-free alternatives give a creamy texture and a hint of nutty richness to your beverage, enhancing the overall enjoyment level. Nut milk is especially popular among people searching for a dairy alternative without sacrificing smoothness.

Choose unsweetened types to preserve control over the sweetness of your smoothie. The delicate nutty undertones match the earthiness of the greens, resulting in a well-balanced and pleasing mix.

4. Green Tea: The Energizing Warm-up

Green tea serves as an invigorating overture to your green smoothie symphony, providing an antioxidant boost as well as a light caffeine rush. Brewed green tea enhances the taste profile while offering possible health advantages. It's an excellent choice for people looking to integrate a delicate tea flavor into their beverage.

Prepare the green tea ahead of time and let it cool before adding it to your smoothie. This liquid base option adds a subtle layer to your symphony, giving each drink a refreshing and exhilarating sensation.

Selecting and Preparing Your Liquid Base: Creating Harmony with Glass

Choosing the proper liquid basis is essential for generating a pleasant green smoothie. The freshness and quality of your liquid help to enhance the overall attractiveness and health advantages of your beverage. Here are some guidelines to help you create the ideal harmony:

1. Freshness Matters

Use fresh, high-quality liquids to improve the flavor of your smoothie. Avoid utilizing drinks that have been sitting for a long time.

2. Gradual Addition

While mixing, gradually add the liquid until the desired consistency is achieved. This allows you to adjust the thickness of your smoothie based on your preferences.

3. Experimentation is Key

Feel free to experiment with various liquid bases to find your favorite flavor profile. Mix & combine to discover the precise balance that suits your taste buds.

Finally, the liquid foundation serves as the unsung conductor, bringing together the many tastes of your green smoothie symphony. Whether you choose the pure hydration of water, the tropical serenade of coconut water, the creamy crescendo of nut milk, or the energetic overture of green tea, each option adds a distinct flavor to your cup.

So, let your blender create this symphony of liquid and greens, and drink your way to a healthier, more vibrant self. The route to a nutrient-dense, tasty green smoothie is a joyful exploration of nutritious ingredients and intelligent decisions that benefit your health. Cheers to your ongoing quest to create green smoothies that are both delicious and healthy!

Healthy Fats As Your Green Smoothie Allies

In the quest to create the ultimate green smoothie, the attention has shifted to healthy fats - the hidden heroes that not only improve the texture of your mix but also provide critical elements to support your overall health. Understanding the significance of these good fats in your smoothie, like leafy greens, is essential for creating a delicious and nutritious combination.

1. Avocado: The Creamy Marvel

Avocado, frequently complimented for its creamy texture, enters the smoothie scene as a versatile and nutrient-dense ally. Avocados not only provide a rich smoothness to your mix, but they also contain heart-healthy monounsaturated fats. These fats not only improve the smoothness of your smoothie, but they also promote cardiovascular health.

Avocado is a great option for people looking for a creamy feel without dairy. Simply peel and pit the avocado before adding it to your blender to turn your green smoothie into a velvety masterpiece with a burst of healthy fats.

2. Chia Seeds and Flaxseeds: Omega-3 Boosters

Chia seeds and flaxseeds, little but formidable, are potent companions that add a boost of omega-3 fatty acids to your green smoothie. These essential fats are crucial for maintaining heart function and lowering inflammation in the body. Furthermore, chia seeds and flaxseeds are high in fiber, which promotes digestive health and contributes to a sense of fullness.

To add these seeds to your smoothie, simply sprinkle a spoonful or two before mixing. The seeds absorb moisture, thickening it and imparting a satisfying crunch to your beverage.

3. Nut Butter (Almond, Peanut, etc.): A Protein-Rich Indulgence

Nut butter, such as almond and peanut butter, provides delicious pleasure to your green smoothie while also providing protein and healthy fats. Almond butter, high in monounsaturated fats, promotes heart health, whilst peanut butter delivers a delicious protein boost.

When choosing nut butter, look for those with no added sweeteners or excessive salt. Adding a dollop of your favorite nut butter to the blender adds a creamy richness and nutty taste that complements the greens and fruits in your smoothie.

Discovering Your Ideal Green Smoothie Blend

Experimentation, like with leafy greens and fruits, is essential for creating a well-balanced green smoothie. Finding the appropriate balance of healthy fats, greens, and fruits allows you to customize your mix based on your taste preferences and nutritional goals. Whether you like the creamy magnificence of avocados, the omega-3 boost of chia or flaxseeds, or the protein-packed delight of nut butter, the alternatives are endless.

Tips for Success When Incorporating Healthy Fats into Your Smoothie

1. Fresh Avocado

Choose ripe avocados for the most creaminess. Before you put the avocado in your blender, peel and pit it.

2. Chia seed or flaxseed

Before mixing your smoothie, sprinkle in a spoonful of chia seeds or powdered flaxseeds. Allow the seeds to soak in liquid to create a thicker consistency.

3. Nut butters

Add a dollop of your favorite nut butter for a creamy and decadent finish. To balance tastes and nutritional content, keep portion sizes in check.

Finally, healthy fats play a critical part in improving your green smoothie experience. Whether it's the creamy wonder of avocados, the omega-3 boost from chia or flaxseeds, or the protein-packed delight of nut butter, these buddies improve not just the texture but also the nutritional value of your beverage.

Minerals and Vitamins: Your Green Smoothie Allies

As we uncover the secrets to making the ultimate green smoothie, our attention turns to the unsung heroes: minerals and vitamins. These key ingredients are critical in transforming your smoothie from a delicious mix to a health-promoting powerhouse. Join us as we examine the intricacies of combining minerals and vitamins without getting bogged down in figurative language or metaphors.

1. Magnesium, the Silent Regulator

Magnesium, a key element, quietly controls a variety of biological activities, making it an important friend in your green smoothie journey. Magnesium, which is rich in leafy greens such as Swiss chard, helps to maintain muscle and neuron function, a healthy immune system, and a stable heartbeat. The addition of magnesium-rich greens provides nutritional depth to your smoothie, ensuring that your body reaps the benefits of this quiet hero.

2. Potassium, the Electrolyte Stabilizer

Potassium, another necessary element, plays a key role in maintaining electrolyte balance, and Swiss chard provides an excellent supply. This mineral is essential for cardiovascular health, muscular function, and fluid balance. Incorporating potassium-rich greens into your smoothie is a natural method to support these important biological functions, which contribute to overall health.

3. Vitamins A, K, and C: Antioxidant Trio

Leafy greens, such as kale, produce a symphony of vitamins that function as antioxidants, shielding your body from oxidative stress. Vitamin A promotes visual health, vitamin K is necessary for bone health, and vitamin C strengthens the immune system. Together, these vitamins provide a strong defense against free radicals, resulting in a healthier, more resilient you.

Choosing Fresh Ingredients for Maximum Nutritional Value

The freshness of your components is the key to maximizing the mineral and vitamin content of your green smoothie. Choose vivid, crisp leaves that show no indications of withering or browning. Fresh greens not only improve the flavor, but they also ensure that you get the most nutritional value from these nutrient-dense companions.

Preparation: Creating a Nutrient Symphony

After you've carefully picked your leafy greens, the preparation is a simple but important step. Thoroughly wash the leaves to eliminate contaminants and maintain nutritional integrity. Removing tough stems, especially from kale and Swiss chard, can result in a smoother texture in the final mix.

As you combine these nutrient-dense greens, see them turn from lowly leaves to a nutrient-rich miracle. Experimentation can help you achieve the ideal combination that meets both your taste sensibilities and your nutritional goals. Consider blending different greens to create a symphony of tastes, enabling minerals and vitamins to dance together in your green elixir.

In conclusion, minerals and vitamins are the hidden heroes who turn your green smoothie into a nutrient-dense elixir. Whether it's the quiet regulator, magnesium, the electrolyte stabilizer, potassium, or the antioxidant triad of vitamins A, K, and C, each nutrient is essential for your health. Freshness is essential, and experimentation is required to realize the full potential of these nutritious friends.

The blending step is where your team comes together. The blender, like a well-coordinated move on the field, transforms your ingredients into one coherent entity. The coach is responsible for transforming individual players into a successful team, ensuring that every component contributes to the overall success of your green smoothie.

Experimenting with different combinations is similar to fine-tuning your team's strategy. You may change the component ratio to meet your taste preferences and nutritional goals. Perhaps you want a more tropical vibe, so add additional pineapple. Perhaps you want an extra boost of antioxidants, so you add more berries.

The beauty is in adapting your team to your specific needs. To summarize, building the ideal green smoothie is similar to gathering a dream squad of nutritious buddies. Each component has a unique purpose, from the robust greens providing the basis to the creamy banana contributing texture, the flavor-packed berries, the spicy pineapple, and the hydrating drink guaranteeing the proper consistency.

The blending process serves as a coach, transforming individual players into a successful team. By experimenting and changing the ingredients, you may create a green smoothie that not only tastes delicious but also provides a significant nutritional boost. So collect your ingredients, press the mix button, and let your nutritious dream team work their magic!

Discover The Best Fit for your Smoothie Adventure

Searching for the best blender to suit your smoothie adventure is like exploring a large environment with several options. Let's simplify this investigation by eliminating sophisticated vocabulary and metaphors.

Imagine yourself in a store full of blenders, each with its unique set of features and capabilities. This plethora of possibilities may appear intimidating at first, but don't worry; we're here to walk you through the process of selecting the ideal fit for your smoothie-making needs.

Learning the Fundamentals: What Is a Blender?

Before we go into the realm of blenders, let's define what a blender is. A blender is a kitchen gadget that mixes and blends diverse components, resulting in a smooth and uniform texture. It is generally made up of a container with sharp revolving blades driven by an electric motor.

Blender Types

1. Countertop Blenders

These blenders are classic and strong, commonly found on kitchen counters. They're adaptable, strong, and ideal for a variety of jobs, including smoothie manufacturing.

Pros: Strong blending abilities, huge capacity, and frequently comes with many speed options.

Cons: Takes up counter space and may be too strong for certain users.

2. Personal Blenders

Personal blenders are compact and practical, making them ideal for individual servings. They frequently come with portable cups that function as drink containers.

Pros: Space-saving, simple to use and clean, great for individual servings.

Cons: Smaller capacity; power may be limited.

3. Immersion Blenders

Also known as hand blenders are handheld devices having blades at the end. They are submerged directly in the components for mixing.

Pros: Simple to use, ideal for blending in pots or bowls, and typically easy to clean.

Cons: While not as powerful as countertop blenders, they are acceptable for specialized applications.

Key Features to Consider: What is Important in a Blender?

1. Power

The power of a blender is measured in watts. Higher watts often indicates higher blending power.

Consideration: For smoothies, a blender with at least 500 watts is generally plenty.

2. Capacity

The volume that a blender can hold is referred to as its capacity. Consider how many servings you'd like to prepare at once.

Consideration: Personal blenders are ideal for single servings, whilst countertop blenders are better suited for bigger amounts.

3. Ease of Cleaning

Think about how simple it is to clean the blender, especially if you use it regularly.

Consideration:

Dishwasher-safe components or blenders with detachable blades might make cleaning easier.

Choosing Your Perfect Match: Decision Factors

1. Your requirements

Consider your unique demands. Do you make daily smoothies for yourself, or do you require a blender for a variety of culinary tasks?

2. Budget

Create a budget depending on your requirements. There are great blenders available at a variety of prices.

Finally, navigating the world of blenders requires recognizing your tastes and demands. Whether you choose a countertop powerhouse, a tiny personal blender, or a multipurpose immersion blender, each has its benefits. Consider the aspects that are most important to you, and let your smoothie journey lead your decision. Cheers to finding your ideal blender mate!

Practical Blending Techniques for Smooth, Palatable Results

Starting the adventure of creating the ideal smoothie is similar to becoming a gourmet artist in your kitchen. However, achieving that immaculate blend entails more than simply throwing items into a blender; it takes a symphony of practical skills to create a smooth, delicious masterpiece.

Your trusted blender is a kitchen partner with a lot of mixing possibilities. Imagine it as a magical wand that turns raw components into a delicious elixir. Whether it's a countertop pitcher with powerful blades or a compact cup for on-the-go convenience, the basic idea is the same: combine your selected ingredients into a harmonious mix.

Choosing the Right Ingredients: Building Blocks

1. **Leafy Greens:** They not only give your smoothie a brilliant green color, but they also provide a variety of critical nutrients.

Tip: For a smoother mix, carefully wash the greens and remove any stiff stems before blending.

2. **Fruits:** Fruits not only enhance the flavor, but they also provide natural sugars.

Tip: Using frozen fruits improves texture and chill factor, adding a refreshing touch to your mix.

3. **Healthful Fats:** Adding healthy fats like avocado, chia seeds, or flaxseeds to your smoothie can increase its creaminess and satiety.

Tip: Use in moderation; a little goes a long way in adding texture without overwhelming the mix.

4. Liquid Base: The liquid foundation, whether it's water, milk, yogurt, or coconut water, acts as a blending conductor, ensuring that all components combine smoothly.

Tip: Begin with a little quantity and progressively adjust while mixing to get the desired consistency.

Practical Blending Techniques: How-To Guide

1. Layering Ingredients

Imagine constructing a taste skyscraper, beginning with the liquid foundation at the bottom and progressing to layers of greens, fruits, and any extra components. This deliberate stacking creates an equal mix.

Tip: By ordering your components in this careful sequence, you may avoid blade jams and get a smoother blend.

2. Begin Slow, Gradually Increase Speed

Imagine this as a slow crescendo in a musical composition. Begin blending at a slow speed to break up bigger parts, then gradually raise the speed to get a seamless, smooth composition.

Tip: Patience is a virtue while mixing; hurrying can interrupt the rhythm and produce uneven textures.

3. Pulse Technique

Pulsing allows you to channel your inner DJ by combining brief bursts of music to create a rhythmic pattern. This procedure eliminates overheating and guarantees a perfect blend.

Tip: Pulse when you meet bigger pieces; it's like giving your components a dance break as they progressively break down.

4. Tilt and Tap

Sometimes substances appear to be trapped. Consider your blender a cooperative partner; tilt or tap lightly to spread ingredients throughout the blades, resulting in a more coordinated mix.

Tip: If there are any obstinate bits, a simple twist and tap can bring your smoothie to perfection.

5. Experiment with texture

Consider your blender to be a flexible instrument with customizable settings. Blend longer for a velvety texture or shorter for a more textured, vibrant look. Adjust to your unique taste preferences.

Tip: Listen to the symphony of blending; a smoother blend is typically accompanied by a softer melody.

Once you've mastered these practical mixing methods, it's time for the big finale. Pour your flavor symphony into a glass or container of your choice. Enjoy the captivating colors and tantalizing perfume flowing from your masterpiece. Remember that the satisfaction of a superb smoothie comes not only from its flavor but also from the creativity involved in its creation. With these strategies at your disposal, you're not simply blending, but creating a smooth, appetizing masterpiece every time.

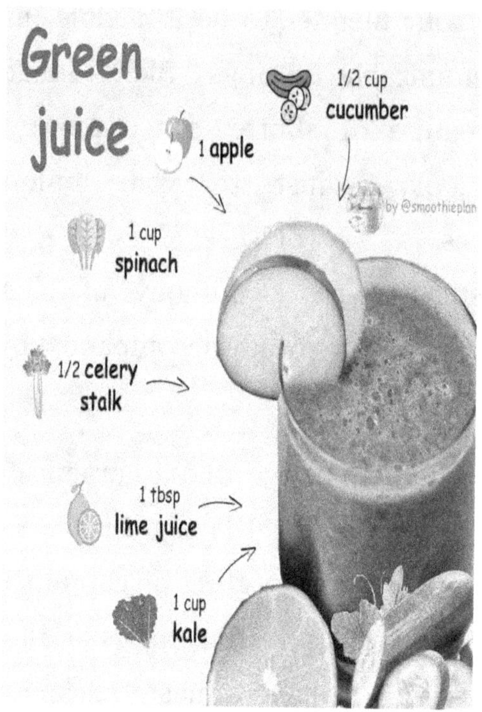

Chapter 6: Getting Started - 30 Days Plan Overview

Starting a 30-day plan is similar to creating a clear blueprint for your goals. Consider it a practical roadmap, breaking down your journey into manageable chores for the following month. This plan acts as your daily roadmap, guiding you toward achievement in a simple and attainable manner.

Consider making a well-structured plan with particular activities for each day. It's a smart technique that ensures you focus on actionable stages and breaks down your broader goal into digestible chunks. Each day's responsibilities serve as stepping stones, eventually guiding you to your objective.

Consider this plan to be a toolbox, with each day providing a distinct tool to help you succeed. By following this plan, you're not overwhelmed by the large picture but are empowered to confront each day's issues efficiently.

As the days pass, you'll notice your improvement, and the small successes will add up to get you closer to your ultimate objective. So, plunge into your 30-day plan with zeal, and let your everyday achievements pave the path for your ultimate success!

Preparation and Planning For The 30-Days Healthy Green Smoothie Plan

Ready to start on a colorful adventure of health and deliciousness? Welcome to "The 30-Day Healthy Green Smoothie Plan," your personalized guide to implementing the power of green smoothies into your daily routine for a month of restored energy, well-being, and vitality. But before you dive headfirst into your blender, let's prepare for success with a strategy as fresh and exciting as the smoothies themselves!

Defining Your "Why"

Before stirring up a storm, pause to identify your distinctive "why."What do you aim to achieve with this 30-day adventure? Do you intend to raise your energy levels, improve digestion, assist weight control, or simply explore delightful new methods to nourish your body? Having a defined objective will keep you motivated and help you adapt your smoothie selections throughout the plan.

Planning Your Pantry

Stocking your kitchen with a varied selection of smoothie components is vital for success. Think of it as constructing a vivid green arsenal! Here are some crucial categories to consider:

Leafy Greens: Kale, spinach, collard greens, romaine lettuce - these nutritious powerhouses form the backbone of your green revolution. Start with 2-3 handfuls of each smoothie and experiment with different varieties.

Fruits: Berries, bananas, apples, pears, mangoes - offer sweetness, taste, and important vitamins. Choose frozen or fresh, based on availability and choice.

Fiber Champions: Chia seeds, flaxseeds, oats — these fiber fighters keep you feeling full and improve digestion. Start with 1-2 teaspoons each smoothie and increase gradually.

Hydration Heroes: Cucumber, celery, watermelon - these watery wonders contribute to fluid intake and keep things running smoothly.

Liquid Foundation: Water, unsweetened almond milk, coconut water — use your chosen foundation for the desired consistency and nutritious profile.

Building Your Blend

Now for the fun part — designing your unique smoothie creations! Here are some suggestions for making nutrient-packed blends:

Start with the Greens:

Use 2-3 handfuls of your preferred leafy greens as the base for every smoothie.

Mix and Match Fruits:

Experiment with different combinations of fruits for taste and diversity. Berries are a particularly strong source of antioxidants.

Don't Forget Fiber:

Include 1-2 tablespoons of chia seeds, flaxseeds, or oats for satiety and digestive health.

Hydration Boost: Add ½ cup of cucumber, celery, or watermelon for an extra hydration kick.

Liquid Love: Choose your chosen liquid foundation (water, almond milk, etc.) to get the ideal consistency and modify for extra nutrient profiles.

Spice it Up (Optional): Fresh ginger, turmeric, lemon, or mint can give a zing of taste and added health benefits.

Creating Your Schedule

Decide how you want to add green smoothies into your day. Will they be a regular breakfast, a pleasant afternoon snack, or a post-workout recovery drink? Choose a plan that matches your lifestyle and guarantees you enjoy the smoothies regularly throughout the month.

Shopping Savvy

Planning your grocery list in advance will save you time and money. Buy frozen fruits and veggies while they're on sale, and consider going for pre-washed greens for ease. Invest in reusable containers for keeping pre-portioned smoothie components, making mixing a snap.

Preparation Pointers

- Wash and cut all fruits and veggies before keeping them in airtight containers.
- Portion out leafy greens and other ingredients in advance for speedy mixing.

- Prepare freezer bags with pre-measured fruit combinations for a grab-and-go option.
- Keep your blender clean and conveniently accessible for regular usage.

Beyond the Blend

Remember, "The 30-Day Healthy Green Smoothie Plan" is simply one component of your total health jigsaw. To completely enhance your well-being, consider these extra practices:

Listen to your body: Don't push yourself to drink a smoothie if you're not feeling it. Adjust ingredients or skip a day if required.

Hydration Hero: Remember to drink lots of water throughout the day, alongside your smoothies.

Move it or Lose it: Incorporate regular physical exercise into your routine for maximum health and well-being.

Mindfulness Matters: Practice mindful eating to relish your smoothies and build a good connection with food.

The 30-day green smoothie regimen is an adventure, not a constraint. There will be days you explore with flavors, find new preferences, and feel the burst of energy from nutritional deliciousness. There can also be days when you desire something else or need a break. The goal is to listen to your body, appreciate the process, and celebrate every step towards a better, happier

Setting Achievable Goals: A Practical Guide for Your 30-Day Green Smoothie Journey

Starting the 30-Day Healthy Green Smoothie Plan is like setting sail on a journey to a better self. Setting realistic goals for this journey is essential, so let's break it down in simple words.

Understanding Realistic Goals for the 30-Day Green Smoothie Plan

Consider reasonable goals as individual milestones on your smoothie adventure. Instead than striving for dramatic improvements, focus on tiny, attainable goals. These goals serve as stepping stones, helping you through the 30-day trip with a sense of accomplishment.

Why Realistic Goals Are Important in Your Green Smoothie Journey

Consider your objectives to be the compass that guides you through this healthy journey. Realistic objectives are important because they help you stay on track without overwhelming you. They work as realistic indicators, allowing you to make steady progress without feeling discouraged.

Setting Your Goals for the 30-Day Challenge

Imagine your objectives as precise locations on a

smoothie map. Rather than a general aim for health improvement, break it down into specific goals. For example, one specific objective may be to consume a nutrient-dense green smoothie every morning during the challenge.

Start Small, Think Big for Your Smoothie Plan

Visualize your aspirations as little seeds that grow into major accomplishments. Begin with little chores, such as including one green smoothie each day. This method positions you for success, making the trip more pleasurable and feasible.

Flexibility in Green Smoothie Goals

Think of your objectives as adjustable plans, similar to a flexible itinerary. Life is dynamic, and circumstances may change. Allowing yourself the opportunity to adapt your smoothie objectives keeps you on track, even if the road changes somewhat.

Tracking Your Green Smoothie's Progress

Consider chronicling your smoothie journey as a simple diary. It's not just about getting to the end of the day, but also about enjoying the little sips in between. Regularly evaluate your progress, recognizing how your daily green ritual helps to your overall well-being.

Celebrating Green Smoothie Milestones

Consider achieving your smoothie objectives as crossing refreshing finish lines. As you move forward, don't forget to rejoice in every achievement. It's like checking off completed chores on your to-do list, acknowledging and rewarding your dedication to a better living.

Use Your Green Smoothie Support System

Visualize your support system as a smoothie crew cheering you on. Share your objectives with friends and family who can inspire you. This support system works as fellow sailors on your adventure, providing encouragement and direction as required.

Adjusting Your Green Smoothie Expectations

Consider altering your expectations as recalibrating your smoothie compass. As you work your way through the difficulty, your perception of what is possible may shift. Be willing to adjust your goals to reflect your evolving taste buds and health goals.

Finally, choosing realistic goals for the 30-Day Healthy Green Smoothie Plan is similar to developing a personalized trip map. It's more than simply finishing the challenge; it's about enjoying the savory journey, savoring the daily sips, and celebrating each health-conscious milestone.

Understanding the relevance of realistic objectives prepares you for a rewarding journey of good change. So, grab your blender, plan your smoothie route, and enjoy the thrill of transforming your green goals into refreshing, attainable accomplishments!

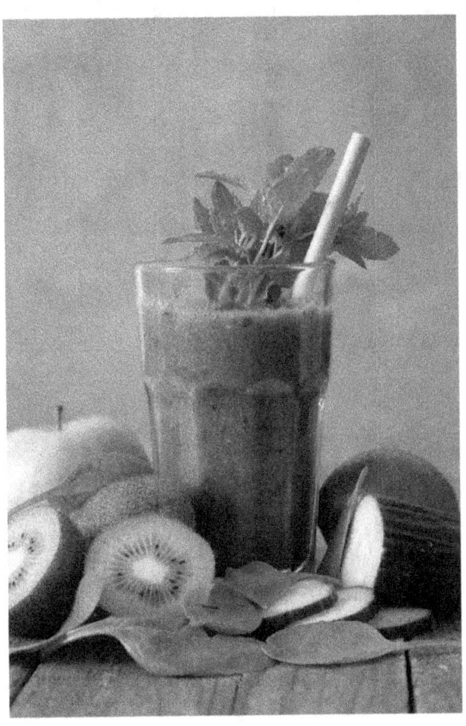

Chapter 7: Day-by-Day Guide

This chapter is your step-by-step manual for the 30-Day Healthy Green Smoothie Plan. Think of it as your daily roadmap, guiding you through the journey. This section breaks down each day, making it easy for you to follow and stay on track. It's like having a friendly companion, providing clear instructions without any complicated language.

The guide ensures you know exactly what to do each day, making the whole process simple and enjoyable. Consider it your go-to resource, offering practical insights for a successful and fulfilling 30-day green smoothie adventure.

Day 1-5: Introducing Green Smoothies

Days 1-5 of your 30-Day Healthy Green Smoothie Plan are like entering a refreshing world of colorful flavors and health benefits. These initial days are all about bringing yourself to the goodness of green drinks. Let's dive into this kickstart phase with simple, useful language, avoiding complicated terms.

Understanding the Introduction to Green Smoothies

Think of Days 1-5 as your smoothie introduction. It's like opening the door to a new, better living. During this time, we focus on introducing your taste buds to the wonderful mix of leafy greens, fruits, and liquid bases that make up your green smoothie.

What's in Your Green Smoothie

Your green smoothie is a mix of fresh greens like spinach or kale, fruits such as berries or bananas, and a liquid base like water or almond milk. This mix promises a tasty and nutrient-packed beverage.

Beginning the Green Smoothie Adventure: Days 1-5 Unveiled

Welcome to the first chapter of your 30-day green

smoothie journey, which promises more than simply nourishment but also a reinvigorated, healthier you. As you begin the first five days, consider this phase not just as a habit, but as the basis for a lifetime change. Let's look at what to expect throughout these fundamental days, including the information, images, and explanations that will walk you through each stage of this revolutionary process.

1. Introduction to Leafy Greens: Unlocking the Nutrient Treasure Chest

Learn about nutritious leafy greens such as spinach, kale, and Swiss chard. Learn about the nutritional advantages of each green, which can help you live a better lifestyle.

Begin by looking at the mild-mannered challenger, spinach. Visualize its vivid, fresh leaves and consider how they contribute to your daily nutrient requirements. Dive further into the minerals it provides, including vitamins A and C for eyesight and immunological support, as well as iron for healthy blood.

Spinach, the Clark Kent of leafy greens, offers a gentle introduction. Consider it the unsung hero of your green smoothie, providing nutritious benefits without overwhelming your taste receptors. Highlight spinach's versatility beyond smoothies, making it an ideal choice for a variety of culinary applications.

2. Harmony with Fruits: Creating a Symphony of Flavors

Try combining leafy greens with fruits such as bananas, berries, and tropical fruits. Discover the delicious and approachable side of green smoothies by embracing the natural sweetness of fruits.

Visualize the rich colors and textures of kale with berries or Swiss chard with tropical fruits. Consider the harmonic combination, resulting in a symphony of tastes in your blender.

Kale, the strong champion, enters the smoothie scene with powerful and earthy flavors. Consider its nutritious richness as it compliments the natural sweetness of fruits, offering a significant health benefit. Explore the diversity of taste combinations to make each sip a memorable experience.

3. Understanding the Liquid Base as the Canvas for Your Creation

Learn about the smoothie's liquid basis, which might be water, coconut water, or almond milk. Recognize how the liquid foundation serves as a canvas, bringing the elements together into a well-balanced symphony.

Think of the liquid base as the unifying ingredient, perfectly mixing greens and fruits into a smooth, drinking masterpiece. Consider the symphony to be composed of water, coconut water, and almond milk, each with its own distinct flavor.

Think of the liquid foundation as the canvas for your smoothie creation. It serves as a backdrop for the brilliant hues of the greens and fruits. Recognize the purpose of each liquid option: water for simplicity, coconut water for natural sweetness, and almond milk for a creamy mouthfeel.

4. Sipping to Holistic Well-Being

Practice mindful drinking to promote overall well-being. Make a link between your green smoothie and a renewed, invigorated lifestyle.

Consider introducing green smoothies into your daily routine: a refreshing start in the morning, a lunchtime pick-me-up, or a post-workout replenishment. Consider the green smoothie to be more than just a drink; it is a partner on your quest to overall well-being.

Green smoothies are about more than simply nutrition; they are about transforming your lifestyle. Imagine your mornings beginning with a green elixir, a lunchtime boost to tackle responsibilities, or a post-workout refill. Understand how mindful sipping promotes a link between what you eat and the rejuvenation it provides to your entire health.

5. Mindful Sips, Wholesome Living: Nourish Your Body and Soul

Practice mindful sipping by appreciating each taste and nutritional benefit. Create a regimen that promotes not only sustenance but also a better, more vibrant version of yourself.

Imagine yourself taking time to savor the color, scent, and flavor of your green smoothie. See how each drink becomes a conscious act that nourishes both your body and your spirit. Imagine the daily practice establishing a foundation for a healthy, lively existence.

The core of the first five days is careful drinking. It's more than just drinking; it's a conscious act of nurturing your body and spirit. Understand how this habit will serve as a basis for a healthier, more vibrant version of yourself.

Below is the summary that has been explained so far about the first to with day of beginning your green smoothie plan:

Starting Simple:

Visualize these first days as the beginning of a delicious trip. We keep it simple initially, using known ingredients to make the change easy. Basic recipes might include broccoli, banana, and water – a delicious mix that sets the tone for the days ahead.

Building a Routine

Think of making a green smoothie routine as forming a daily habit. During Days 1-5, try to add one green smoothie into your routine. This could be a morning routine, a refreshing afternoon pick-me-up, or even a healthy dessert option.

Tasting and Adjusting

Imagine these opening days as a tasting experience. Sip your green drink and pay attention to tastes. If you find it to be too thick, add more liquid. If you prefer a sweeter taste, try with different veggies. This part is about finding your preferences.

Listening to Your Body

Consider tuning in to how your body reacts. Green smoothies can be energizing, so watch your energy levels and general well-being. This is like having a conversation with your body, knowing what it values.

Celebrating the Start:

Visualize finishing Days 1-5 as crossing the starting line of a healthy path. Celebrate this initial milestone – it's like marking off the first steps towards a lively, healthy lifestyle.

In conclusion, Days 1-5 are your green smoothie start, an introduction to a world of health and taste. The focus is on simplicity, routine-building, and finding what fits your taste buds. These days lay the basis for the exciting and rewarding trip that lies ahead in your 30-Day Healthy Green Smoothie Plan.

Consider green smoothies as your daily vitamin boost. They provide important vitamins, minerals, and antioxidants that help to general well-being. The greens offer fiber for processing, while fruits bring natural sweetness and extra nutrients.

Green smoothies are more than simply a fashionable beverage; they are a powerhouse of health benefits, providing a pleasant and nutritious method to improve your overall well-being. Let's look at the benefits of adopting these bright combinations into your everyday routine.

1. Nutritional Superheroes

- **Vitamins Galore:**

Green smoothies contain vital vitamins A, C, and K from leafy greens, which promote visual health, immunological support, and bone strength.

- **Mineral Boost:**

Ingredients like Swiss chard include nutrients like magnesium and potassium, which help with bone health and electrolyte balance.

2. Weight Control Support

- **Fiber for Satiety:**

Green smoothies with leafy greens and fruits include fiber, which promotes fullness and helps with weight control.

- **Nutritionally Dense and Low in Calories:**

These beverages have a high nutrient-to-calorie ratio, which helps you lose weight while still providing your body with critical nutrients.

3. Gut Health Harmony

Digestive Support:

Green smoothies include fiber, which promotes healthy digestion, prevents constipation, and supports a balanced gut microbiota.

Hydrating Bonus:

The liquid foundation in green smoothies aids in hydration and general digestive function.

4. Antioxidant Armor

Combat Oxidative Stress:

Leafy greens, such as kale, contain antioxidants that reduce inflammation and protect cells from harm.

Cellular Defense:

Regular antioxidant consumption helps the body defend against chronic illnesses and promotes overall cellular health.

5. Energy Elixir

Natural Energy Boost:

Fruits include vitamins, minerals, and natural sugars that deliver a long-lasting energy boost without the crash of sugary drinks.

After-Workout Refuel:

Green smoothies are a fantastic post-workout snack, restoring nutrients and promoting muscle repair.

6.Hydration with Flavor

Refreshing Hydration:

Green smoothies are a pleasant alternative to plain water that promotes fluid intake and overall hydration.

Flavorful Variety:

You may enjoy a variety of flavors while being hydrated by combining vegetables, fruits, and liquid bases.

7. Clear and Glowing Skin

Hydrated Complexion:

Proper hydration and nutrition intake promote clearer, more radiant skin.

Anti-Inflammatory Properties:

Antioxidants included in green smoothies may help reduce skin inflammation and promote a healthy complexion.

8. Blood Sugar Balance

Balanced Sugar Absorption:

Fiber in leafy greens reduces sugar absorption and promotes stable blood sugar levels.

Suitable for diabetics:

Green smoothies can be diabetic-friendly if carefully prepared using low-sugar fruits and vegetables.

9. Whole-Body Detox

Supports Natural Detoxification:

Nutrients and antioxidants support the body's natural detoxification processes, reducing toxins and waste.

Liver and Kidney Support:

Green smoothies include chemicals that promote liver and kidney function, which is essential for proper detoxification.

10. Heart Health

Cholesterol Management: Green smoothies' fiber and antioxidants promote heart health by managing cholesterol levels.

Blood Pressure Support:
Potassium-rich compounds help to maintain normal blood pressure.

Incorporating green smoothies into your daily routine is more than just a fad; it's a delicious path to a healthier, more vibrant you. Sip, enjoy, and let the green elixir improve your overall health !

Days 6-15: Boosting Detox with Green Power

As you move into Days 6-15 of your 30-Day Healthy Green Smoothie Plan, imagine moving into a phase where the focus changes to accelerating detoxification through the power of green goodness.

Understanding The Accelerated Detox Phase

Think of Days 6-15 as a boost for your body's natural cleaning processes. It's like opening the windows to let in fresh air, cleaning your system from within. During this step, we increase the detoxifying qualities of your green smoothies.

Powerful Ingredients for Detox

Your green smoothies during this time will include ingredients known for their detoxifying effects. Let's delve into the world of powerful ingredients that make a detox green smoothie not only delicious but also a robust cleanser for your system.

1. Leafy Greens (Spinach, Kale)
Visualize leafy greens as the superheroes of your detox journey. Spinach and kale, rich in vitamins and minerals, play a pivotal role in supporting your body's natural detox pathways. These greens contribute to overall health while aiding in the elimination of toxins.

2. Cucumber

Envision cucumber as a hydrating companion in your green smoothie adventure. Its high water content not only refreshes your palate but also supports kidney function, actively participating in the elimination of toxins from your system.

3. Celery

Imagine celery as the crisp addition that adds more than just a satisfying crunch. This humble vegetable contributes to hydration and detoxification.

Including celery in your green smoothie not only enhances its flavor but also brings added benefits to your body's cleansing process.

4. Lemon

Picture lemon as the detox powerhouse that adds a zesty twist to your smoothie. Packed with vitamin C, lemons support liver function and aid the body in eliminating waste. Including lemon in your green smoothie not only enhances its flavor profile but also boosts its detoxifying properties.

5. Ginger

See ginger as the warm and soothing element in your green concoction. Beyond its distinctive flavor, ginger serves as a natural anti-inflammatory, contributing to a thorough detoxification process. It aids digestion and adds a therapeutic touch to your green smoothie experience.

6. Chia Seeds

Envision chia seeds as tiny yet mighty detox warriors. These seeds provide a generous dose of fiber, promoting healthy digestion. As you sip your green smoothie, chia seeds work to flush out toxins, contributing to a more efficient cleansing process for your body.

7. Coconut Water

Imagine coconut water as the tropical hydrator that elevates your green smoothie to a delightful experience. Apart from its delicious taste, coconut water replenishes electrolytes, supporting your body during the detox journey. It adds a touch of tropical flair while ensuring you stay hydrated.

Crafting your detox green smoothie is akin to assembling nature's detox toolkit in your blender. Picture the vibrant colors and flavors blending into a nourishing elixir. As you sip on this powerful concoction, imagine each ingredient working synergistically to cleanse, replenish, and revitalize your body. The journey to a healthier, more energized you begins with every sip of your potent green smoothie detox. Cheers to vibrant well-being!.

The Health Benefits of Green Smoothie Detox

Going on a green smoothie detox is more than simply drinking a delicious beverage; it's a transforming experience for your entire health. Incorporating a regular detox practice into your routine encourages continuing cleaning and improves overall health.

Let's look at the amazing benefits that detoxing with green smoothies may offer to your body:

1. Elimination of Toxins

Assume your body as a canvas, and toxins are unwelcome brushstrokes. Green smoothie detox works like an eraser, assisting your body in eliminating accumulated toxins. The potent mix of substances boosts natural detoxification processes, resulting in a cleaner interior environment.

2. Improved Digestion

Think of your digestive system as a well-coordinated symphony. Green smoothies, which are high in fiber and contain nutrients like leafy greens and chia seeds, act as a conductor, enabling a smooth digestion process. This improves digestion and allows for more effective nutrient absorption.

3. Enhanced Energy Levels

Imagine your energy levels as a flickering flame. Green smoothie detox adds fuel to the fire by giving an abundance of vitamins, minerals, and antioxidants. This infusion of important nutrients combats weariness, leaving you feeling refreshed and rejuvenated.

4. Enhanced Hydration

Consider your body to be a growing garden, with water serving as the life-giving substance. Green smoothies, which frequently include hydrating components such as cucumber and coconut water, help to maintain proper hydration. This is critical for sustaining biological functioning, aiding detoxification, and fostering healthy skin.

5. Weight Management

Visualize your path as a continuous rise. Green smoothies, especially when combined with a well-balanced diet, can help with weight management. The fiber content improves fullness, which helps to curb cravings and contributes to a healthy weight.

6. Glow Skin

Consider your skin as a mirror of your inside health. Green smoothie detox boosts antioxidants and moisture, resulting in a more luminous complexion. The vitamins and minerals in these smoothies feed your skin from within, resulting in a healthy glow.

7. Balanced Blood Sugar

Think of your blood sugar levels as a tightrope walk. Green smoothies made with carefully selected ingredients can help to maintain stable blood sugar levels. The fiber and nutrient-rich composition helps to control glucose absorption, which promotes overall metabolic health.

8. Immune System Support

Think of your immune system as a protective barrier for your body. Green smoothies, which include immune-boosting elements such as vitamin C, help to build a strong immune system. Regular ingestion can add an extra layer of protection against common ailments.

Embracing the advantages of a green smoothie detox extends beyond the flavor; it is about nourishing your body and cultivating a holistic feeling of well-being. So, raise your glass to a healthier, more energized you with each drink of your green smoothie mixture!

Experimenting with Green Combinations

Consider trying different green mixtures as a culinary journey. Mix and match veggies, fruits, and liquids to discover a mix that both detoxifies and delights your taste buds. This step is about finding combinations that connect with you.

Everyday Detox Routine

Incorporating a regular detox practice into your routine encourages continuing cleaning and improves overall health. Imagine adding a daily detox drink as building a healthy habit.

Aim to enjoy at least one green detox drink each day during this time. It's like having a daily routine that actively adds to your overall well-being. Consider the following basic yet effective measures to make detoxification a daily practice:

1.Morning Hydration

Start your day with a glass of warm water laced with lemon. This procedure not only hydrates your body after a night's sleep, but it also aids digestion and speeds up your metabolism.

2. Green Smoothie Boost

Introduce a nutrient-dense green smoothie into your regular regimen. This delightful combination mixes leafy greens, fruits, and a liquid base to deliver critical vitamins and minerals while also assisting in cleansing.

3. Herbal Tea Interlude

Throughout the day, drink herbal teas recognized for their cleansing effects. Dandelion tea, for example, promotes liver function, whilst ginger tea improves digestion and lowers inflammation.

4. Mindful Movement

Add mild workouts or stretching to your everyday regimen. Physical exercise increases circulation, which aids in the clearance of toxins from the body.

4. Hydrating Infusions

Infuse your water with detoxifying ingredients like cucumber, mint, or berries. These natural ingredients not only improve the flavor but also have additional cleaning properties.

5. Evening Epsom Salt Bath

Relax in the evening with an Epsom salt bath. This exercise not only relaxes muscles but also aids in detoxifying through the skin, resulting in a comfortable night's sleep.

6. Digital Detox Before Bedtime

Prioritize a digital detox before bedtime. Limit your screen time to improve your sleep quality and enable your body to focus on its natural detoxifying activities at night.

Adding these daily detox practices to your routine is a proactive method to help your body's natural cleansing systems. Consistency in these routines enables a continual and lasting approach to detoxification, which benefits your general health.

Listening to Your Body's Detox Signals

Going on a green smoothie detox journey is more than simply drinking a nutritious combination; it's about recognizing the subtle signals your body gives as it detoxifies. Let's look at the symphony of detox signals your body may send during this cleaning journey.

1. Increased Hydration

Signs of increased hydration include feeling thirstier than normal. As your body removes pollutants, it needs more water to wash them out. Increased thirst indicates that your system is reacting to this demand.

2. Frequent Urination

Frequent bathroom breaks indicate increased urination. Your kidneys help you eliminate waste. An increase in toilet trips suggests that your kidneys are busy removing toxins from your body.

3. Clearer Skin

Significant improvement in skin tone. Detoxification can help you have clearer skin by allowing your body to eliminate toxins that might cause acne or other skin problems. A glowing complexion is a good indicator of the detox process.

4. Boost in Energy Levels

Feeling more energetic and alive. As your body eliminates pollutants, you may experience an increase in energy levels. This indicates that your system is working more efficiently, and you are receiving the benefits of increased nutritional absorption.

5. Improved Digestive Function

Less bloating or digestive pain. Detoxifying your body typically results in better digestion. Reduced bloating or pain implies that your digestive system is absorbing nutrients more efficiently.

6. Changes in Bowel Movements

Increased frequency in bowel movements. A cleanse can improve bowel motions, increasing regularity. Changes in stool consistency or frequency might indicate your body's efforts to remove waste.

7. Enhanced Mental Clarity

Improved concentration and mental clarity. Detoxifying your body can improve cognitive performance. Improved mental clarity and attention indicate that your brain is benefiting from lower toxin levels.

8. Elevated Mood

Feeling energized and positive. Detoxification can improve mood by lowering inflammation and increasing the release of feel-good neurotransmitters. A more optimistic view is a beneficial reaction to the detox process.

9. Reduced Cravings for Unhealthy Foods

Lower desire for processed or unhealthy foods. As your body cleanses, you may notice a decrease in cravings for sugary or processed meals. This adjustment in desires indicates that your taste preferences are aligning with healthier options.

10. Balanced Sleep Patterns

Better sleep quality and patterns. Detoxification promotes general body functioning, including sleep. If you're sleeping more deeply or have improved sleep patterns, it's a good sign for your general health.

Listening to these detox signals helps you to understand your body's unique responses and enjoy the good changes that occur during your green smoothie detox journey. As the detox symphony plays, savor each note and let the harmony of well-being emerge.

Celebrating the Detox Progress

Think of completing Days 6-15 as hitting a milestone in your detox process. Celebrate the progress you've made — it's like recognizing the positive changes happening within your body as you commit to a better, cleaner lifestyle.

Celebrating detox wins with more energy, cleaner skin, and improved mental clarity. Celebrate waking up refreshed, getting comments on your glowing skin, and experiencing emotional harmony. Mark better gut function, decent sleep, and controlled cravings as milestones.

Each good change represents your body's response to the detoxification process. By acknowledging your accomplishments, you reaffirm your commitment to a healthy lifestyle and generate enthusiasm for continuing improvement on your detox journey.

Conclusion: Green Power Detox

In conclusion, Days 6-15 put you into the green power detox phase, a time of increased cleansing and rejuvenation. This section emphasizes the detoxifying potential of your green smoothies, adding vegetables known for their cleansing qualities. Cheers to improving your detox journey and feeling the refreshing effects of green power!

Day 16-30: Focusing on Weight Loss

As you stride into the final part of your 30-Day

Healthy Green Smoothie Plan (Days 16-30), imagine this phase as a focused journey toward weight loss through the vibrant world of green smoothies. Let's dig into the facts using clear and simple language, keeping away from complicated terms .

Understanding the Weight Loss Focus

Think of Days 16-30 as a focused effort towards achieving weight loss goals. It's like fine-tuning your method to harness the full potential of green smoothies in losing extra weight.

Ingredients Tailored for Weight Loss

During this time, your green smoothies will include ingredients specially chosen to support weight loss. Imagine leafy greens like spinach or kale, metabolism-boosting fruits such as berries or oranges, and hydration-enhancing drinks like water or herbal tea.

The choices you make when making green drinks with the goal of helping you lose weight are very important. Let's look at the parts of a green smoothie that is full of nutrients and can help you lose weight without using fancy words or images.

1. Leafy Greens: the best way to lose weight - Think of healthy greens like spinach and kale as the ones who will help you lose weight. They make you feel full without making you gain weight because they are low in calories and high in fiber. These greens also give you minerals and vitamins that are good for your health.

2. Fruits That Speed Up Your Metabolism

Think about adding foods that are known to speed up the metabolism. Berries, oranges, and apples fall into this group. These foods contain compounds that may improve calorie burning and add to general metabolic health, helping in your weight loss efforts.

3. Low-Calorie Fruits for Sweetness

Consider using low-calorie foods like berries and citrus fruits to add sweetness without extra sugars. This ensures a tasty experience without compromising your weight loss goals. You can think of these fruits as the natural sweeteners that go well with your green drink.

4. Hydration-Enhancing Liquids

Think of water, herbal tea, or coconut water as the drinks that improve hydration in your green smoothie. Staying hydrated is important for weight loss, helping digestion, reducing appetite, and supporting general metabolic processes. These drinks are like the clean, refreshing base of your weight-loss-friendly mix.

5. Protein-Packed Additions

Visualize adding protein sources like Greek yogurt, chia seeds, or protein powder into your green drink. Protein promotes satiety, making you feel full for a more extended time. This addition is like the building block that sustains your energy and supports muscle health during your weight loss journey.

6. Healthy Fats for Satiety

Consider adding a source of healthy fats, such as avocado or a spoonful of nut butter, to your green drink. These fats add to a feeling of fullness, avoiding unnecessary snacking. Think of them as the pleasant elements that keep hunger at bay during your weight loss efforts.

7. Green Tea Boost

Imagine adding green tea into your drink for an additional metabolism boost. Green tea includes catechins, which may help in burning fat. This addition is like the natural stimulant that supports your weight loss journey.

8. Fiber-Rich Ingredients

Picture including fiber-rich components like flaxseeds or psyllium husk. Fiber improves digestive health and adds to the feeling of fullness. These ingredients act like the gentle sweepers that help your body in its natural cleaning process during weight loss.

In conclusion, tailoring your green smoothie ingredients for weight loss includes a careful selection of nutrient-dense elements that support your goals. Imagine these ingredients as a team working together to provide important nutrients, promote fullness, and add to a satisfying and effective weight loss trip.

Weight Loss Benefits of Green Smoothies

Visualize the weight loss phase as a relationship between your body and nutrient-dense green drinks. These beverages aid weight loss by providing necessary nutrients, boosting feelings of fullness, and supporting metabolism. It's like having a natural partner in your weight loss journey.

Starting a weight loss journey may be a fulfilling endeavor if it is addressed with equilibrium and simplicity. Leafy greens, such as spinach and kale, are a great way to start losing weight since they are high in nutrients and satisfy your hunger without adding extra calories.

Imagine your smoothie to be a symphony of fruits, with citrus, apples, and berries all collaborating in perfect harmony. In addition to their inherent sweetness, these fruits contribute essential vitamins, minerals, and antioxidants that improve general health and create a colorful backdrop for your weight reduction efforts.

Water, herbal tea, or coconut water are your vital hydration companions; they produce the cool streams that sustain and balance your weight reduction efforts. Include protein sources like as Greek yogurt or chia seeds. These are like adding sturdy gears to your weight reduction machine; they will keep you feeling full and energized for a longer period of time.

Imagine if during your weight reduction journey, satiating foods like avocado or nut butter are made of healthy fats. These fats serve as reassuring cushions, enhancing your pleasure and reducing the need for mindless munching.

Create your green smoothie mindfully, approaching each item as a planned step in your diet plan. By acknowledging and appreciating minor accomplishments along the road, you can make your trip successful, sustainable, and fulfilling.

Creating Your Daily Weight Loss Ritual

Starting a weight reduction journey takes a persistent and conscientious attitude. Consider adding a daily weight loss smoothie as building a healthy habit. This routine ensures you regularly provide your body with nutrient-packed, low-calorie options that help to weight loss. It's like making a daily ritual that actively helps your weight loss journey.

1. Morning Hydration

Start your day by hydrating your body. Consider a pleasant glass of water as a metabolic wake-up call. Hydration stimulates your digestive system and improves your general well-being.

2. Green Smoothie Kickstart

Imagine a nutrient-dense green smoothie as the foundation of your morning routine. Add leafy vegetables, fruits, and a protein source. This smoothie is a healthful and pleasant breakfast that sets a good mood for the day.

3. Mindful Meal Planning

Consider preparing your meals with forethought. Consider eating a variety of lean meats, healthy grains, and colorful veggies. Consider each meal an opportunity to provide your body with essential nutrients.

4. Snack Smartly

Consider nutritious snacks like almonds, yogurt, or fresh fruits as allies throughout the day. These snacks satisfy hunger and give long-lasting energy, avoiding the temptation of less nutritional alternatives.

5. Stay Active

Include exercise in your everyday routine. It might be a brisk stroll, a short workout, or even stretching. Physical activity boosts your metabolism and promotes general well-being.

6. Maintain Hydration Throughout the Day

Visualize hydration as a daily theme. Carry a water bottle and take regular sips. Staying hydrated aids digestion and regulates appetite.

7. Reflect and Relax

Consider pausing to reflect on your accomplishments and problems. To handle stress, use relaxation techniques such as deep breathing and meditation. This mental health component is essential for a comprehensive weight reduction strategy.

8. Early meal and Wind Down

Consider eating a light meal. Give your body time to digest the meal before going to bed. Consider settling down with a relaxing routine to indicate to your body that it's time to rest.

Finally, this daily weight reduction practice is intended to be both simple and practical. Each component helps to create a balanced and sustainable strategy to weight loss. By visualizing these stages, you may transform your weight reduction journey into a series of focused and manageable daily actions.

Understanding Your Body's Weight Loss Signals

When you want to reduce weight, think of it as a nice conversation with your body. Imagine your body notifying you whether it's hungry or full. Pay attention to these cues and allow them determine when and how much you eat. Consider it as a collaboration between you and your body.

Consider tuned in to the cues - perhaps your stomach growls a bit or feels comfortably full. This creates a pleasant connection with your body, making weight loss feel more like a natural knowledge of what your body requires rather than a set of severe restrictions.

Simply said, losing weight is a journey in which you and your body collaborate, making decisions based on this amicable conversation. It's like working with your body to get healthier and happier.

Celebrating the Weight Loss Achievements

Think of completing Days 16-30 as hitting a major milestone in your weight loss journey. Celebrate the progress you've made — it's like recognizing the positive changes happening within your body as you commit to a better, more balanced lifestyle.

In conclusion, Days 16-30 mark the weight loss end of your 30-Day Healthy Green Smoothie Plan, focusing on meeting your weight loss goals with the help of nutrient-dense green smoothies. This phase tailors ingredients to support weight loss, stressing a balanced approach and celebrating your

successes. Cheers to reaching your weight loss goal
and enjoying a healthier, more energetic you!

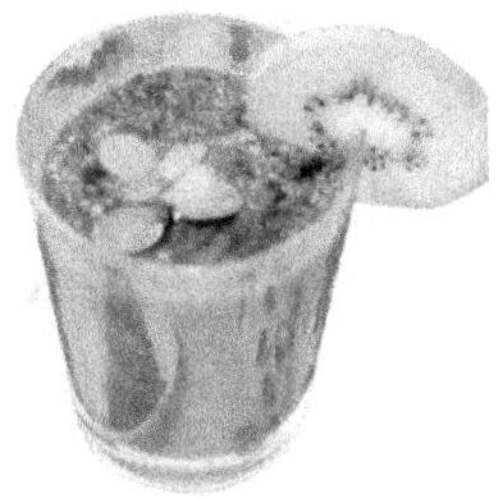

Chapter 8: Recipes and Meal Plans

In this chapter, we'll look at practical and tasty green smoothie recipes, as well as simple meal planning. Discover a selection of delicious combinations that not only satisfy your taste senses but also help you achieve your health objectives.

From refreshing morning blends to fulfilling meal replacements, these recipes make it easy to incorporate green smoothies into your daily routine. The accompanying meal plans guide you through a well-rounded and nutrient-dense diet, assuring a pleasant path toward a healthy living.

Simple Green Smoothie Recipes

Simple Green Smoothie Recipes are easy-to-follow steps for making delicious and healthy green smoothies. These recipes typically involve blending a mixture of leafy veggies, fruits, liquid bases, and possible add-ins like nuts or seeds. The goal is to provide a straightforward guide for people, even those with minimal cooking skills, to introduce healthy green beverages into their daily routine.

The materials are widely found in grocery stores, and the preparation methods are meant to be quick and simple. These recipes aim to make the process of incorporating green smoothies into your diet approachable, enjoyable, and, most importantly, helpful to your general well-being. Whether you're looking for a refreshing start to your day or a nutrient-packed snack, simple green smoothie recipes offer a handy and tasty answer.

Breakfast Green Smoothie Recipes

1. Beginner's Bliss

Ingredients:

- 1 cup spinach
- 1 banana
- 1 cup water

Preparation:

- Blend all ingredients until smooth.

Nutritional Value:

- Calories: 120

- Fiber: 3g

- Vitamin A: 56% DV

- Vitamin C: 22% DV

2. Berry Boost

Ingredients:

- Handful of kale

- A cup of mixed berries (strawberries, blueberries)

- 1/2 cup almond milk

Preparation:

- Put all the ingredients in the blender and blend until well mixed.

Nutritional Value:

- Calories: 150

- Fiber: 5g

- Vitamin K: 68% DV

- Antioxidants: High

3. Tropical Delight

Ingredients:

- 1/2 cup pineapple chunks

- 1/2 mango

- 1 cup spinach

- 1 cup coconut water

Preparation:

- Blend until smooth.

Nutritional Value:

- Calories: 160

- Vitamin B6: 15% DV

- Electrolytes: Replenished

4. Citrus Zing

Ingredients:

- 1 orange (peeled)

- 1 cup kale

- 1/2 cup Greek yogurt

- 1/2 cup water

Preparation:

- Blend until creamy.

Nutritional Value:

- Calories: 140

- Protein: 10g

- Vitamin C: 90% DV

5. Green Protein Punch

Ingredients:

- 1 scoop protein powder

- Handful of spinach

- 1/2 banana

- 1 cup almond milk

Preparation:

- Blend until the protein powder dissolves.

Nutritional Value:

- Calories: 200

- Protein: 25g

- Iron: 12% DV

6. Creamy Avocado Dream

Ingredients:

- 1/2 avocado

- 1 cup spinach

- 1/2 cup pineapple

- 1 cup coconut milk

Preparation:

- Blend until creamy.

Nutritional Value:

- Calories: 180

- Healthy Fats: 14g

- Vitamin E: 10% DV

7. Blueberry Bliss

Ingredients:

- 1 cup blueberries

- Handful of kale

- 1/2 cup Greek yogurt

- 1/2 cup water

Preparation:

- Blend until smooth.

Nutritional Value:

- Calories: 160

- Antioxidants: High

- Probiotics: Present

8. Spinach Banana Crunch

Ingredients:

- 1 cup spinach

- 1 banana

- 1/4 cup granola

- 1 cup water

<u>Preparation:</u>

- Blend until desired consistency.

<u>Nutritional Value:</u>

- Calories: 180

- Fiber: 4g

- Iron: 8% DV

9. Peanut Butter Powerhouse

<u>Ingredients:</u>

- 2 tablespoons peanut butter

- Handful of kale

- 1 banana

- 1 cup almond milk

<u>Preparation:</u>

- Blend until creamy.

<u>Nutritional Value:</u>

- Calories: 250

- Protein: 9g

- Healthy Fats: 20g

10. Carrot Cake Smoothie

Ingredients:

- 1/2 cup carrots (shredded)

- 1/4 cup oats

- 1/2 teaspoon cinnamon

- 1 cup coconut water

Preparation:

- Blend until the oats are well incorporated.

Nutritional Value:

- Calories: 130

- Beta-Carotene: High

- Fiber: 5g

Enjoy these nutrient-packed breakfast green smoothies to energize your mornings!

Green Smoothie Lunch Recipes

1. Mediterranean Green

Ingredients:

- 1 cup spinach

- 1/2 cucumber (peeled)

- 1/4 cup feta cheese

- 1/4 cup olives

- 1 tablespoon olive oil

Preparation:

- Blend until smooth.

Nutritional Value:

- Calories: 180

- Healthy Fats: 14g

- Vitamin K: 85% DV

2. Protein-Packed Veggie Blend

Ingredients:

- 1 cup kale

- 1/2 cup Greek yogurt

- 1/2 cup cherry tomatoes

- 1/4 cup almonds

- 1 cup water

Preparation:

- Blend until creamy.

Nutritional Value:

- Calories: 220

- Protein: 15g

- Vitamin C: 40% DV

3. Avocado & Chickpea Fiesta

<u>Ingredients:</u>

- 1/2 avocado

- 1/2 cup cooked chickpeas

- Handful of cilantro

- 1/2 lime (juiced)

- 1 cup coconut water

<u>Preparation:</u>

- Blend until well combined.

<u>Nutritional Value:</u>

- Calories: 240

- Healthy Fats: 16g

- Fiber: 10g

4. Spicy Spinach Gazpacho

<u>Ingredients:</u>

- 1 cup spinach

- 1/2 cup cucumber

- 1/2 bell pepper

- 1/4 cup red onion

- 1 tablespoon hot sauce

<u>Preparation:</u>

- Blend until gazpacho consistency.

Nutritional Value:

- Calories: 150

- Vitamin A: 45% DV

- Hydration: Boosted

5. Quinoa Kale Fusion

Ingredients:

- 1 cup kale

- 1/2 cup cooked quinoa

- 1/4 cup pineapple chunks

- 1/2 cup almond milk

Preparation:

- Blend until smooth.

Nutritional Value:

- Calories: 200

- Protein: 8g

- Iron: 10% DV

6. Tomato Basil Elegance

Ingredients:

- 1 cup basil leaves

- 1 cup cherry tomatoes

- 1/4 cup Parmesan cheese

- 1/2 lemon (juiced)

- 1 cup water

Preparation:

- Blend until basil is finely chopped.

Nutritional Value:

- Calories: 160

- Vitamin C: 30% DV

- Calcium: 15% DV

7. Tropical Kale Fusion

Ingredients:

- 1 cup kale

- 1/2 cup mango

- 1/2 cup pineapple

- 1/4 cup coconut flakes

- 1 cup coconut water

Preparation:

- Blend until tropical bliss.

Nutritional Value:

- Calories: 220

- Vitamin C: 70% DV

- Electrolytes: Replenished

8. Caesar Salad Greenie

<u>Ingredients:</u>

- 1 cup romaine lettuce

- 1/4 cup Caesar dressing

- 1/4 cup croutons

- 1/4 cup Parmesan cheese

- 1 cup water

<u>Preparation:</u>

- Blend until Caesar salad consistency.

<u>Nutritional Value:</u>

- Calories: 180

- Fiber: 5g

- Vitamin K: 60% DV

9. Beet Berry Boost

<u>Ingredients:</u>

- 1/2 cup beets (cooked)

- 1 cup mixed berries

- 1/4 cup Greek yogurt

- 1 cup water

<u>Preparation:</u>

- Blend until vibrant color achieved.

<u>Nutritional Value:</u>

- Calories: 200

- Antioxidants: High

- Probiotics: Present

10. Greek Goddess Green

<u>Ingredients:</u>

- 1 cup spinach

- 1/4 cup Greek yogurt

- 1/2 cucumber (peeled)

- 1/4 cup kalamata olives

- 1 tablespoon olive oil

<u>Preparation:</u>

- Blend until goddess-worthy.

<u>Nutritional Value:</u>

- Calories: 160

- Protein: 6g

- Healthy Fats: 12g

These lunch green smoothies are not only delicious but also packed with nutrients to fuel your afternoon!

Dinner Green Smoothie Recipes

1. Spinach & Garlic Elegance

Ingredients:

- 1 cup spinach

- 1/2 avocado

- 1/2 clove garlic

- 1 tablespoon lemon juice

- 1 cup water

Preparation:

- Blend until garlic is finely mixed.

Nutritional Value:

- Calories: 160

- Healthy Fats: 12g

- Vitamin C: 20% DV

2. Cauliflower & Berry Bliss

Ingredients:

- 1 cup cauliflower (steamed)

- 1/2 cup mixed berries

- 1/4 cup almond butter

- 1 cup almond milk

Preparation:

- Blend until creamy texture.

<u>Nutritional Value:</u>

- Calories: 220

- Fiber: 8g

- Antioxidants: High

3. Broccoli & Blueberry Delight

<u>Ingredients:</u>

- 1 cup broccoli (steamed)

- 1/2 cup blueberries

- 1/4 cup Greek yogurt

- 1 cup water

<u>Preparation:</u>

- Blend until smooth consistency.

<u>Nutritional Value:</u>

- Calories: 180

- Protein: 10g

- Vitamin K: 40% DV

4. Zucchini & Mango Fusion

<u>Ingredients:</u>

- 1/2 cup zucchini

- 1/2 cup mango

- 1/4 cup cashews

- 1 cup coconut water

Preparation:

- Blend until tropical delight.

Nutritional Value:

- Calories: 200

- Healthy Fats: 14g

- Vitamin C: 60% DV

5. Sweet Potato & Spice Symphony

Ingredients:

- 1/2 cup sweet potato (baked)

- 1/2 teaspoon cinnamon

- 1/4 teaspoon nutmeg

- 1/4 cup oats

- 1 cup water

Preparation:

- Blend until warm and spiced.

Nutritional Value:

- Calories: 220

- Fiber: 6g

- Vitamin A: 150% DV

6. Asparagus & Apple Zing

Ingredients:

- 1 cup asparagus (steamed)

- 1/2 green apple

- 1/4 cup walnuts

- 1 cup water

Preparation:

- Blend until refreshing zing.

Nutritional Value:

- Calories: 190

- Healthy Fats: 15g

- Fiber: 7g

7. Cabbage & Kiwi Cooler

Ingredients:

- 1 cup cabbage

- 1/2 kiwi

- 1/4 cup hemp seeds

- 1 cup coconut water

Preparation:

- Blend until a refreshing cooler.

Nutritional Value:

- Calories: 210

- Protein: 9g

- Omega-3 Fatty Acids: 6g

8. Carrot & Almond Creaminess

Ingredients:

- 1 cup carrots (steamed)

- 1/4 cup almonds

- 1/2 banana

- 1 cup almond milk

Preparation:

- Blend until creamy texture.

Nutritional Value:

- Calories: 180

- Healthy Fats: 10g

- Vitamin A: 220% DV

9. Bell Pepper & Pear Pleasure

Ingredients:

- 1 cup bell pepper

- 1/2 pear

- 1/4 cup chia seeds

- 1 cup water

Preparation:

- Blend until a pear-infused delight.

Nutritional Value:

- Calories: 190

- Fiber: 8g

- Antioxidants: Abundant

10. Eggplant & Pineapple Paradise

Ingredients:

- 1 cup eggplant (grilled)

- 1/2 cup pineapple

- 1/4 cup coconut flakes

- 1 cup coconut water

Preparation:

- Blend until tropical paradise.

Nutritional Value:

- Calories: 230

- Healthy Fats: 12g

- Vitamin C: 45% DV

These dinner green smoothies are not only savory but also provide a healthy, nutritious way to end your day!

Balanced Meal Suggestions

Balanced meal ideas refer to meal plans that include a range of nutrients in appropriate amounts to support general health. These meals generally contain a mix of important food types, such as proteins, carbohydrates, fats, vitamins, and minerals, ensuring a well-rounded and nutritious diet.

The goal is to make meals that add to a balanced diet, meeting the body's nutritional needs for best performance. This method helps people keep energy levels, support bodily functions, and promote general well-being. Here are some balanced meal suggestions that cover different food groups:

1. Grilled Chicken Salad

- Grilled chicken breast (lean protein)
- Mixed greens (vegetables)
- Cherry tomatoes (vegetables)
- Cucumber slices (vegetables)

- Olive oil vinaigrette (healthy fats)

2. Quinoa Bowl

- Cooked quinoa (whole grains)

- Black beans (protein and fiber)

- Avocado slices (healthy fats)

- Salsa (vegetables)

- Grilled veggies (vegetables)

3. Salmon with Sweet Potato and Broccoli

- Baked salmon filet (omega-3 fatty acids)

- Roasted sweet potato (complex carbohydrates)

- Steamed broccoli (fiber and vitamins)

- Lemon for flavor

4. Vegetarian Stir-Fry

- Tofu or tempeh (plant-based protein)

- Brown rice (whole grains)

- Stir-fried mixed vegetables (bell peppers, broccoli, carrots)

- Soy sauce and ginger for flavor

5. Mediterranean Chickpea Salad

- Chickpeas (protein and fiber)

- Cherry tomatoes (vegetables)

- Cucumber chunks (vegetables)

- Feta cheese (calcium and flavor)

- Olive oil dressing (healthy fats)

6. Green Smoothie and Greek Yogurt Parfait

- Green smoothie (leafy greens, fruits, liquid base)

- Greek yogurt (protein)

- Granola (whole grains)

- Berries (antioxidants)

7. Grilled Chicken Wrap with a Side of Greens

- Grilled chicken strips (lean protein)

- Whole-grain wrap (fiber)

- Mixed greens and tomatoes (vegetables)

- Hummus or avocado spread (healthy fats)

8. Salmon Quinoa Bowl

Salmon cooked by baking or grilling (rich in omega-3 fatty acids).

- Quinoa (whole grains)

- Steamed broccoli and carrots (vegetables)

- Lemon-tahini dressing (flavor and healthy fats)

9. Vegetarian Buddha Bowl

- Chickpeas or tofu (plant-based protein)

 - Brown rice (whole grains)

 - Roasted sweet potatoes (complex carbohydrates)

- Sautéed kale or spinach (leafy greens)

10. Turkey and Vegetable Stir-Fry

- Ground turkey (lean protein)

- Stir-fried mixed vegetables (bell peppers, snap peas, carrots)

- Brown rice or cauliflower rice (fiber)

- Soy-ginger sauce (flavor)

These balanced meals ensure you're not only getting the benefits of green smoothies but also enjoying a variety of nutrients from different food groups. Adjust the portions based on your dietary needs and preferences.

Remember to adjust portion sizes based on your individual dietary needs and goals. These meals provide a good balance of macronutrients (protein, carbohydrates, and fats) and micronutrients (vitamins and minerals)

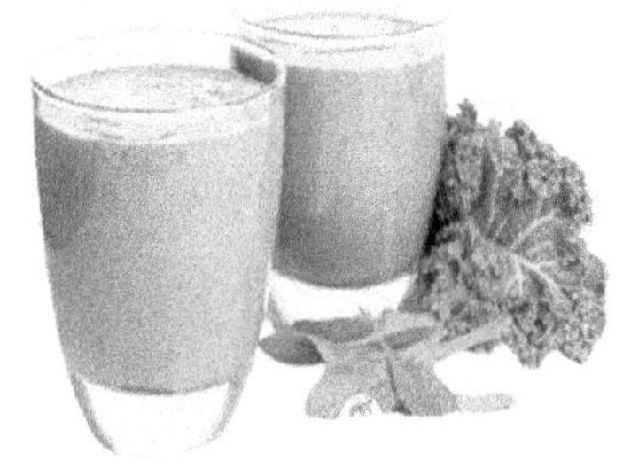

Chapter 9: Incorporating Exercise

Incorporating exercise during the 30-Day Green Smoothie Plan is a key component to maximize the overall health benefits of your journey. This involves integrating physical activity into your daily routine to complement the nutritional aspects of the plan. Activities can range from brisk walks and yoga to more intense workouts, depending on your fitness level and preferences.

Exercise contributes to cardiovascular health, enhances metabolism, and aids in weight management, synergizing with the goals of the green smoothie plan. Additionally, it enhances mental well-being by diminishing stress and uplifting mood. The combination of nutrient-rich smoothies and regular exercise creates a holistic approach to wellness, ensuring you're not only nourishing your body from within but also keeping it active and resilient.

Suitable Exercises for Beginners

Incorporating physical exercise into your routine during the 30-Day Green Smoothie Plan is a crucial aspect of supporting general health and well-being.

For newbies, the focus should be on engaging, approachable workouts that gradually build strength, flexibility, and endurance. Here's a thorough guide to suitable workouts designed for those starting their fitness journey.

1. Walking: The Foundation of Movement

Walking is a low-impact workout that serves as an excellent starting point for newbies. It needs no special equipment, making it available to almost everyone. Begin with short walks and gradually increase the length as your health improves. Walking not only adds to physical health but also offers mental ease and stress reduction.

2. Bodyweight Exercises: Building Strength

Bodyweight exercises are effective for growing strength without the need for weights or tools. Examples include squats, lunges, push-ups, and crunches. These exercises involve multiple muscle groups, building general strength and stability. Start with a few repetitions and gradually increase as your power improves.

3. Yoga: Enhancing Flexibility and Relaxation

Yoga is a flexible workout that blends physical postures with focus and controlled breathing. It improves flexibility, balance, and rest. Many beginner-friendly yoga poses are available online, allowing you to practice in the comfort of your home. Yoga is not only helpful for physical health but also supports mental well-being by reducing stress and improving mood.

4. Cycling: Low-Impact Cardio

Cycling is a low-impact physical workout that is gentle on the joints. Whether using a stationary bike or riding outdoors, it offers an effective way to improve cardiovascular health. Start with shorter workouts and gradually raise the length and intensity. Cycling is not only a great workout but also a useful way of transportation.

5. Swimming: Full-Body Workout

Swimming provides a comprehensive workout for the entire body and is gentle on the joints. It uses different muscle groups and improves cardiovascular fitness. If you have access to a pool, swimming laps or even water exercises can be excellent choices for newbies. The buoyancy of the water lessens impact, making it ideal for people with joint issues.

6. Stretching: Improving Flexibility

Incorporating stretching movements into your routine helps flexibility and range of motion. Stretching can be done as a solo activity or as part of a warm-up and cool-down practice. Focus on major muscle groups, keeping each stretch for 15-30 seconds. Stretching helps avoid injury, improves posture, and increases general mobility.

7. Dance: Fun Cardiovascular Activity

Dancing is not only a fun and enjoyable sport but also an effective aerobic exercise. Whether following dance workout videos or taking a dance class, it elevates the heart rate and improves stamina. Dance allows for self-expression and is a great way to stay busy without feeling like you're doing a regular workout.

8. Resistance Bands: Adding Variety to Workouts

For beginners looking to add resistance training, resistance bands offer a flexible and portable choice. They provide resistance during workouts, helping build power and tone muscles. Resistance band workouts can target various muscle groups and are good for people of different fitness levels.

Tips for Getting Started

- Consult with a healthcare worker before starting a new workout plan, especially if you have any current health conditions.

- Begin with workouts that match your current fitness level and gradually improve.

- Listen to your body and make changes as needed to avoid damage.

- Stay consistent and make exercise a normal part of your practice.

In conclusion, incorporating suitable exercises into your 30-Day Green Smoothie Plan improves the general effect on your health. Whether you choose walks, bodyweight movements, yoga, riding, swimming, stretching, dance, or resistance training, finding things that you enjoy will make keeping active a sustainable and fun part of your lifestyle. Remember, the goal is growth, not perfection.

Enhancing Results through Physical Activity

Getting more exercise during the 30-day healthy green smoothie plan can help you reach your goals.

To live a healthy life, adding physical exercise helps you reach your goals faster and better, and it works perfectly with the 30-Day Healthy Green Smoothie

Plan. Consuming nutrient-dense green drinks is only one part of this all-around method; it also includes taking care of your physical health.

Benefits That Work Well together

The 30-Day Healthy Green Smoothie Plan is all about giving your body a daily amount of nutrient-rich green smoothies, which will help you lose weight and clean. These benefits work together to make a strong synergy when combined with regular physical exercise. It has an unmatched effect on blood health, metabolism, and general fitness.

Weight Management Made Better

Working out is a great way to lose weight, and it works even better when you drink green shakes. Smoothies help you get the nutrients you need in a controlled way, but exercise is the most important thing because it burns calories. The mixture forms a harmonious equation, supporting a healthy balance between energy intake and expenditure for lasting weight control.

Boosting Energy Levels

Engaging in physical exercise increases the release of endorphins, generally known as "feel-good" chemicals. This increase in positive neurochemicals supports the energy-boosting qualities of the green smoothies. The result is a heightened sense of vitality, making daily chores more doable and promoting an active lifestyle.

Cognitive Enhancements

Both the 30-Day Healthy Green Smoothie Plan and daily physical exercise add to brain well-being. The nutrient-rich greens in the smoothies support brain health, giving important vitamins and minerals. Simultaneously, exercise improves brain function, improving memory and mental clarity. This dual-pronged method ensures a thorough boost to brain health.

Stress Reduction and Mental Clarity

Modern lives often bring about worry and mental fatigue. Green smoothies, with their variety of nutrients, and physical exercise serve as stress busters. The smoothies provide a nutritional buffer against stress, while exercise acts as a physical release, relaxing strain and boosting mental focus. This combo helps in creating a balanced and resilient mental state.

Strategies for Synergy

To harness the full potential of combining the 30-Day Healthy Green Smoothie Plan with physical exercise, certain tactics can be adopted. Incorporate exercises that match with personal tastes and fitness levels. This could range from short walks to more intense workouts based on individual skills.

Setting achievable goals for both diet and fitness is important. Establishing a habit that smoothly combines green smoothies and physical exercise into daily life ensures continuity. This tandem method is about building lasting habits that add to long-term health.

In conclusion, improving results through physical exercise within the framework of the 30-Day Healthy Green Smoothie Plan provides a harmonious symphony of well-being. The complementary nature of these aspects gives a complete approach to health, covering physical exercise, cognitive well-being, and stress relief. As you start on this journey, recognize the power of synergy between nutrient-packed green elixirs and the invigorating effects of physical exercise – a powerful recipe for a healthier and more vibrant you.

Chapter 10: Overcoming Challenges

In the context of the 30-Day Healthy Green Smoothie Plan, overcoming hurdles refers to tackling different barriers or difficulties that people may have while following the plan. These challenges could include adjusting to new tastes, managing social situations where dietary choices differ, dealing with cravings for specific foods, adjusting to changes in digestion, finding time for preparation, and overcoming other obstacles that may arise during the transition to a healthier lifestyle.

The objective is to develop practical ways to make the strategy more achievable and sustainable. Navigating the 30-Day Healthy Green Smoothie Plan has distinct obstacles. Overcoming these problems needs commitment, organization, and a good attitude. Here's how to overcome typical obstacles:

1. Taste Adjustment

Getting used to the taste of green smoothies might be difficult, especially if you aren't used to eating leafy greens. Begin with gentler greens, such as spinach, and gradually introduce stronger-flavored alternatives. Experiment with different fruit combinations to discover one that matches your taste.

2. Social Situations

Managing social situations when unhealthy food options are abundant can be difficult. Share your health objectives with your friends and family. Bring your green smoothie to events and make informed choices from the available alternatives. Focus on the social component rather than just the meal.

3. Cravings

It's natural to experience cravings for unhealthy snacks or meals. To fulfill your appetite, make healthful green smoothies. Include a mix of fruits and greens to keep the tastes interesting. When cravings occur, choose healthy snacks and eat in moderation.

4. Time Constraints

Balancing the responsibilities of daily life with the creation of green smoothies might be difficult. To make the blending process go more smoothly, prepare components ahead of time, such as cleaning and portioning greens. Consider creating larger quantities so you may have smoothies ready to go throughout the week.

5. Varietal Boredom

It's normal to get tired with the same old green smoothie choices. Embrace diversity by experimenting with different greens, fruits, and liquid bases. Explore recipes and get creative with your ingredients. Experimenting with different tastes keeps things interesting.

6. Lack of Support

Making the trek without a support system might be difficult. Seek encouragement from friends, family, and online networks. Share your experiences, learn from others, and celebrate your accomplishments together. Building a support system can help boost motivation..

A

7. Digestive Adjustments

Increased fiber consumption is often associated with digestive abnormalities. Slowly include fiber-rich components into your smoothies to allow your digestive system to adjust. Stay hydrated to promote proper digestion.

8. Energy Swings

During the adjustment period, it is normal to have energy swings. Recognize that your body may require time to adapt. To keep your energy levels up, prioritize sleep, remain hydrated, and eat nutrient-dense meals.

9. Picky Eaters

Encouraging toddlers or fussy eaters to join the green smoothie adventure might be difficult. Involve children in the preparation process by enabling them to select ingredients. Experiment with various flavors until you find combinations that appeal to their palates.

10. Sustainability

Maintaining the green smoothie habit after 30 days might be challenging. Create a post-plan habit by including green smoothies into your everyday life. Set achievable goals, develop a range of dishes, and concentrate on the long-term health advantages.

11. Ingredient Availability

Finding fresh greens may be difficult depending on your region. Investigate local markets, frozen choices, or try starting a tiny indoor garden.

12: Exercise Adherence

Maintaining a consistent fitness program can be challenging. Select activities that you love, begin with moderate durations, and progressively build intensity. Find an exercise companion to help you stay motivated.

13. Budget Constraints

Healthy ingredients may be seen as pricey. Plan your meals, shop in bulk, and try local, seasonal vegetables. Look for cost-effective solutions that do not compromise nutrition.

14. Physical Fatigue

Fatigue while exercise is normal, especially if you are new to regular physical activity. Listen to your body, get enough rest, and consider doing low-intensity workouts like yoga on rest days.

15. Nutritional Knowledge

Understanding nutritional content might be intimidating at first. Educate yourself progressively. Use credible sources, visit experts, and concentrate on the fundamentals of a healthy diet.

Individuals embarking on the 30-Day Healthy Green Smoothie Plan will have a more comprehensive toolset to handle any roadblocks with these additional challenges and answers. Participants may make their experience more pleasurable and effective by addressing these challenges with proactive solutions.

Dealing with Cravings

Navigating cravings is a frequent problem when starting a better lifestyle, particularly during the 30-Day Healthy Green Smoothie Plan. Understanding the underlying reasons of cravings and using appropriate solutions will considerably help you manage and overcome them.

Understanding Cravings

Cravings are intense desires or urges for specific foods or flavors, often triggered by emotional, psychological, or physiological factors. These compelling feelings can lead individuals to seek out and consume particular foods to satisfy the perceived need or desire.

Understanding cravings involves recognizing the various factors influencing them, such as emotional states, nutritional deficiencies, or habits. It's crucial to distinguish between genuine hunger and cravings to make informed dietary choices and maintain a balanced and healthy lifestyle.

Emotional triggers, habits, dietary deficits, and hormone variations are all common causes of cravings. Identifying the unique nature of cravings is critical for developing focused interventions.

1. Emotional Awareness

Cravings are not limited to physical hunger, but can also be connected to emotions. Stress, boredom, and even enjoyment may cause cravings. Increasing emotional awareness and finding alternate methods to cope with feelings, such as practicing mindfulness or taking up a hobby, can help remove the emotional link to specific meals.

2. Balanced Nutrition

Nutrient deficits can lead to cravings. It is critical to have a balanced diet that includes macronutrients (proteins, fats, and carbs) as well as micronutrients (vitamins and minerals). Green smoothies, which contain a range of fruits, vegetables, and liquid bases, offer a nutrient-dense choice for meeting fundamental nutritional requirements.

3. Hydration

Dehydration might be perceived as hunger, resulting in unwanted cravings. Staying hydrated with water or herbal teas might help to reduce false hunger signals and promote overall health.

4. Gradual Modifications

Abrupt dietary changes might cause severe cravings. Gradually introducing healthier options and making long-term changes to eating patterns allows the body and mind to adjust more smoothly, lowering the risk of excessive cravings.

5. Mindful Eating

Mindful eating is staying present throughout meals, appreciating each mouthful, and paying attention to hunger and fullness indicators. This strategy promotes a better connection with food and reduces impulsive cravings.

6. Healthier Options

Substituting healthful snacks for unhealthy ones is a sensible method. Having a variety of nutritious snacks on hand, such as fruits, almonds, or yogurt, can help you fulfill cravings while staying on track with your health objectives.

7. Balanced Foods

Ensuring that each meal is well-balanced, with a variety of proteins, healthy fats, and carbs, helps boost fullness and minimize cravings between meals.

8. Planning and Preparation:

Creating a meal plan and preparing items ahead of time might help you avoid making poor food choices at the last minute. This proactive strategy reduces exposure to attractive items that might cause cravings.

9. Sleep Quality

Inadequate sleep can upset hormonal balance, resulting in increased desires, particularly for sweet or high-calorie foods. Prioritizing adequate sleep is critical for overall health and successful desire management.

10. Seek Help

Discussing urges with a friend, family member, or a support group may give both motivation and accountability. Sharing experiences and methods can provide crucial insights and inspiration in difficult situations.

Dealing with cravings effectively requires a multifaceted approach that includes self-awareness, nutritional knowledge, and mindful activities. Individuals may better manage cravings by adding these tactics into the 30-Day Healthy Green Smoothie Plan, resulting in a sustained and joyful road to greater health.

Managing Social Situations

Managing social situations while following the 30-Day Healthy Green Smoothie Plan requires finding a fine balance between achieving health goals and engaging in social activities. Here's a guide to efficiently managing social settings while following this plan:

1. Communicate your Choices

Tell your friends and family about your dedication to living a better lifestyle. Tell them about your green smoothie adventure and how it has improved your health. Clear communication helps to manage expectations and garner support.

2. Bring a Green Smoothie

If you're attending a party or celebration, bring your own green smoothie. Not only does this provide you with a nutritional alternative, but it also introduces others to the delightful and healthful world of green smoothies.

3. Select Wisely Among Available Options

When confronted with limited healthy options in social settings, make decisions based on information Choose salads, lean proteins, and other nutritional alternatives when they are available.

Focus on portion management and enjoying the tastes of healthier options.

4. Plan Ahead

Plan your meals around upcoming social events. Before heading out, drink a pleasant green smoothie to limit your chances of indulging in unhealthy foods or overeating.

5. Stay Hydrated

In social circumstances, water may be a helpful ally. Staying hydrated might help you regulate your appetite and avoid mindless munching. Consider drinking a glass of water or herbal tea in between mingling and snacking.

6. Be Aware About Alcohol Consumption

Alcoholic drinks can increase calorie intake and lead to bad eating habits. If you decide to drink, do it in moderation and pick lighter options such as wine or spirits with calorie-free mixers.

7. Practice Moderation

Enjoy your social activities without feeling deprived. Instead of fully shunning delectable pleasures, practice moderation and relish lesser servings. Balance is essential.

8. Seek Support

Discuss your health objectives with friends and family during the social gathering. Having someone aware of your commitment might give encouragement and assistance in navigating any obstacles.

9. Concentrate on the Social Aspect

Make social events more on the people and the experience rather than the food. Engage in chats, activities, and enjoy each other's company. This can minimize the emphasis on eating and result in a more satisfying experience.

10. Remember Your Why

Remind yourself of the reasons you started the 30-Day Healthy Green Smoothie Plan. Whether it's better health, more energy, or weight control, keeping your objectives in mind can help you stay committed.

Effectively managing social circumstances is an essential component of living a healthy lifestyle. Using these tactics, people may confidently handle social gatherings, enjoy the company of others, and stay on track with their health objectives during the 30-Day Healthy Green Smoothie Plan.

Chapter 11: FAQ Section

A FAQ section addresses frequently asked issues about the 30-Day Healthy Green Smoothie Plan, providing clarification and assistance for those participating in the program. This section seeks to anticipate answer questions about preparation, dietary elements, probable problems, and post-plan maintenance.

It is a useful resource for participants, providing practical insights and answers to frequent difficulties, resulting in a more seamless and educated experience throughout the green smoothie journey.

Common Questions Answered

Here are common questions answered in the FAQ section for the 30-Day Healthy Green Smoothie Plan:

1. Q: Can I prepare my green smoothies in advance?

- **A:** Yes, you can prep ingredients ahead to streamline your daily smoothie-making process.

2. Q: How can I adapt the taste of green smoothies to my liking?

- **A:** Experiment with different ingredients, gradually increasing greens, and add natural sweeteners like fruits or honey.

3. Q: Is it okay to use frozen fruits in my smoothies?

- **A:** Absolutely, frozen fruits add convenience and a chilled texture to your green smoothies.

4. Q: What should I do if I find fresh greens hard to come by?

- **A:** Explore local markets, consider frozen options, or even grow a small indoor garden for a fresh supply.

5. Q: How can I maintain consistency throughout the 30 days?

- **A:** Set reminders, create a dedicated smoothie time, and enlist support from family or friends for accountability.

6. Q: Are green smoothies suitable for weight loss?

- **A:** Yes, incorporating nutrient-rich green smoothies can be part of a healthy weight loss plan.

7. Q: What should I do if I experience fatigue during exercise?

- **A:** Listen to your body, ensure adequate rest, and consider incorporating low-intensity exercises like yoga on rest days.

8. Q: How can I deal with social pressures during gatherings?

- **A:** Plan ahead, bring a green smoothie to events, and communicate your health goals with friends and family.

9. Q: Can I explore different recipes for variety?

- **A:** Absolutely, explore diverse combinations of greens, fruits, and liquid bases to keep your plan interesting.

10. Q: Are there alternatives for budget-friendly ingredients?

- **A:** Plan meals, buy in bulk, and explore local, seasonal produce as budget-friendly alternatives.

11. Q: How do I overcome monotony from repetition?

- **A:** Explore diverse recipes, join online communities for ideas, and incorporate different greens, fruits, and liquid bases.

12. Q: Is it possible to continue green smoothies beyond the 30 days?

- **A:** Absolutely, establish a post-plan routine by incorporating green smoothies into your daily life for long-term benefits.

13. Q: Can I consume green smoothies if I have dietary restrictions?

- **A:** Green smoothies are versatile; tailor recipes to accommodate dietary restrictions, and consult a nutritionist if needed.

14. Q: How can I adapt green smoothies for picky eaters or children?

- **A:** Involve them in the preparation process, allowing them to choose ingredients, and experiment with flavors.

15. Q: Should I adjust my green smoothie intake based on my fitness level?

- **A:** Gradually introduce green smoothies and adapt based on your fitness level and energy needs.

16. Q: Can I use green smoothies as meal replacements?

- **A:** While they can be nutritious, it's essential to ensure your overall daily nutritional needs are met.

17. Q: Are there specific greens that are better for beginners?

- **A:** Start with milder greens like spinach and gradually incorporate stronger-flavored options.

18. Q: How can I manage cravings during the plan?

- **A:** Plan satisfying and nutritious green smoothies to curb hunger and opt for healthier snacks when cravings strike.

19. Q: Can I participate if I have a medical condition?

- **A:** Consult with a healthcare professional before starting any dietary changes, including the 30-Day Healthy Green Smoothie Plan.

20. Q: How do I celebrate milestones during the 30 days?

- **A:** Acknowledge achievements, no matter how small, and treat yourself to positive reinforcements outside of food.

These FAQs cover a range of concerns participants might have during their green smoothie journey, offering practical solutions and guidance.

Troubleshooting Guide

A troubleshooting guide is a thorough series of instructions intended to assist individuals in identifying, diagnosing, and resolving difficulties or obstacles that may arise in a certain setting. The troubleshooting guide for the 30-Day Healthy Green Smoothie Plan is designed to help participants overcome typical issues and ensure a successful and pleasurable experience.

Navigating barriers during the 30-Day Healthy Green Smoothie Plan may provide difficulties. This troubleshooting guide tackles frequent concerns and provides practical answers for a smoother journey:

1. Blender Issues

- **Problem:** Uneven blending or trouble processing greens.
- **Solution:** Cut the materials into smaller bits, gradually add the liquid, and keep the blender in good working order.

2. Bland Taste

- **Problem:** Green smoothie lacks taste or is overly weak.

- **Solution:** Experiment with different fruits, modify ratios, and use delicious ingredients like ginger or citrus.

3. Ingredient Separation

- **Problem:** The ingredients in the smoothie are separate.

- **Solution:** Blend the ingredients well, add natural thickeners such as chia seeds, or eat right away.

4. Digestive Discomfort

- **Symptoms** include bloating or digestive difficulties.

- **Solution:** Introduce fiber gradually, remain hydrated, and seek medical attention if symptoms continue.

5. Texture Concerns

- **Problem:** I don't like the texture of the smoothie.

- **Solution:** Vary the component ratios, use various greens, and experiment with other liquid bases.

6. Meal Time

- **Issue:** Unsure of the optimal time to drink the green smoothie.

- **Solution:** Use it as a meal replacement or snack, depending on your tastes and nutritional requirements.

7. Ingredient Allergies

- **Problem:** Allergic responses to certain chemicals.

- **Solution:** Identify allergies, substitute appropriate alternatives, and seek a healthcare professional.

8. Weight Plateau

- **Problem:** Reaching a weight reduction plateau.

- **Solution:** Reconsider portion amounts, integrate diversity, and modify workout regimens to ensure continuous success.

9. Overcoming desires:

- **Challenge:** Managing unhealthy food desires.

- **Solution:** Create delightful green smoothies with a variety of tastes and choose healthy snack options.

10. Hydrating Levels

- **Issue:** Unsure of hydration requirements.

- **Solution:** Keep track of your water intake, especially when you consume more fiber. Stay hydrated.

11. Ingredient Substitutions

- **Issue:** Unavailable or undesirable components.

- **Solution:** Replace with similar options that match your taste preferences and nutritional aims.

12. Travel Challenges

- **Issue:** Difficulty following the plan when traveling.

- **Solution:** Plan ahead, bring portable blenders, and visit local stores for fresh ingredients.

13. Tracing Progress

- **Issue:** The lack of a method for tracking progress.

- **Solution:** Keep a record, take frequent measurements, and celebrate accomplishments to keep motivated.

14. Support System

- **Problem:** Feeling solitary or without support.

- **Solution:** Join online forums, network with like-minded people, and share your experiences to encourage others.

15. Energy Level

- **Issue:** Experiencing energy swings.

- **Solution:** Get enough sleep, eat a well-balanced diet, and try changing the schedule of your green smoothie consumption.

16. Weight Management Plateau

- **Problem:** Difficulty in managing or losing weight.

- **Solution:** Review caloric intake, incorporate more nutrient-dense foods, and reassess exercise intensity and duration.

17. Frozen Ingredients Clumping

- **Problem:** Frozen ingredients sticking together and not blending well.

- **Solution:** Pre-cut frozen items into smaller portions, thaw slightly before blending, and consider using a blender with sufficient power.

18. Smoothie Temperature Preferences

- **Problem:** Unsure about the desired temperature of the green smoothie.

- **Solution:** Experiment with chilled or room temperature options, adapting to personal taste preferences.

19. Handling Leafy Greens

- **Problem:** Difficulty in handling and storing fresh leafy greens.

- **Solution:** Store greens properly in the refrigerator, use within their freshness window, and consider freezing for prolonged use.

20. Unexpected Reactions

- **Problem:** Experiencing unexpected reactions to certain ingredients.

- **Solution:** Identify specific triggers, exclude those ingredients, and consult a healthcare professional for personalized advice.

21. Post-Plan Transition

- **Problem:** Challenges in transitioning to a post-30-day routine.

- **Solution:** Gradually incorporate green smoothies into daily life, maintain a balanced diet, and focus on sustaining positive habits.

22. Serving Size Confusion

- **Problem:** Uncertainty about the appropriate serving size.

- **Solution:** Tailor serving sizes based on individual dietary needs, energy levels, and overall health goals.

23. Family Participation

- **Problem:** Encouraging family members to join the green smoothie journey.

- **Solution:** Involve family in recipe selection and preparation, making the experience enjoyable for all.

24. Understanding Nutrient Labels

- **Problem:** Difficulty in interpreting nutritional information.

- **Solution:** Familiarize yourself with common nutrient labels, seek reliable sources, and consult a nutritionist for guidance.

25. Dealing with Social Pressures

- **Problem:** Navigating social situations that challenge the green smoothie plan.

- **Solution:** Communicate health goals clearly, stand firm in choices, and focus on overall well-being.

26. Combating Mindless Eating

- **Problem:** Falling into the habit of mindless eating.

- **Solution:** Practice mindful eating, savoring each sip, and establishing a designated smoothie time for focused consumption.

27. Managing Liquid Base Quantity

- **Problem:** Difficulty determining the right amount of liquid base.

- **Solution:** Start with smaller amounts and adjust based on desired consistency, gradually finding the perfect balance.

28. Environmental Impact Concerns

- **Problem:** Considering the environmental impact of ingredients.

- **Solution:** Choose local and sustainable options, minimize food waste, and explore eco-friendly packaging alternatives.

29. Enhancing Sleep Quality

- **Problem:** Impact of dietary changes on sleep quality.

- **Solution:** Monitor caffeine intake, maintain a consistent sleep schedule, and prioritize sleep hygiene for improved rest.

30. Celebrating Successes

- **Problem:** Forgetting to celebrate milestones.

- Solution: Acknowledge achievements, reward yourself with non-food treats, and share successes with your support system.

This troubleshooting guide intends to help people on the 30-Day Healthy Green Smoothie Plan overcome obstacles and have a happy and successful experience throughout the trip.

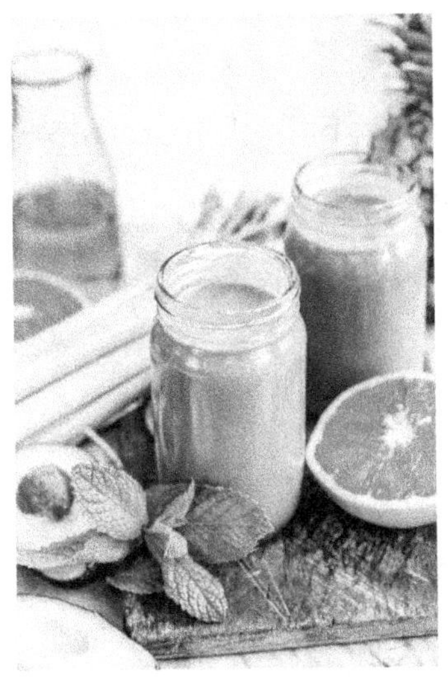

Chapter 12: Tracking Progress

Monitoring your progress is vital during the 30-Day Healthy Green Smoothie Plan. Regularly monitor your progress to keep motivated and make educated decisions. Take note of changes in energy levels, general well-being, and, if relevant, weight reduction.

Keep a notebook, snap photographs, or use an app to track your green smoothie recipes, workout routines, and any obstacles you've conquered. This allows you to celebrate your accomplishments, uncover patterns, and improve your strategy. Accept the transforming process and recognize the plan's beneficial effects on your health and lifestyle.

The Tracking System to Monitor Your Progress

Starting on a 30-day green smoothie journey isn't just about blending delicious drinks; it's a doorway to a vibrant, healthier version of yourself. To make this journey even more rewarding, I present the "30-Day Healthy Green Smoothie Plan Smart Tracking System" – your dynamic progress tracker and smart weight loss device, working hand in hand to lead you through every step of your transformation.

Your Progress Tracker: Your Inner Compass

Imagine your progress tracker as your trusty guide on this 30-day green smoothie adventure, helping you navigate each step with ease and excitement. This as your interactive compass, guiding you through the twists and turns of your green journey:

1. Interactive Calendar

Picture the interactive calendar as your special map for this 30-day green smoothie adventure. It's not just a regular calendar; it's like a fun and colorful guide to track your progress and make each day exciting.

- **Marking Conquered Days**

Every day you conquer on this calendar is like marking a victory on your journey. You can see the days unfold, creating a visual timeline of your green adventure. It's like a colorful canvas where each day tells a part of your story.

- **Personalizing with Recipe Variations**

Want to make it uniquely yours? Imagine having optional checkboxes next to each day, allowing you to track different recipe variations. It's like adding your personal touch to the adventure, making it a vibrant and customized experience.

- **Visualizing Your Green Journey**

The calendar becomes a visual representation of your dedication. It's not just about tracking days; it's about seeing the progress unfold. It's like turning your journey into a colorful and dynamic story, with each day contributing to the bigger picture.

- ## Adding a Splash of Color

Imagine the calendar being a palette of colors, each day a different shade. It's like adding a splash of joy to your journey. The vibrant colors make checking off days a delightful and visually appealing experience.

- ## Creating a Daily Ritual

Checking your interactive calendar becomes a daily ritual, a moment to reflect on your achievements. It's like a pause to appreciate your dedication and acknowledge the steps you've taken towards a healthier lifestyle.

- ## A Motivational Canvas

This calendar isn't just a tool; it's a motivational canvas. It's like a visual reminder of your commitment, encouraging you to keep going. Each marked day is a celebration of progress, turning your calendar into a collection of positive moments.

Daily Habit Tracker

The Daily Habit Tracker can be seen as your checklist for accepting healthy choices during your 30-day green smoothie trip. It's like having a daily companion to help you watch and celebrate not just your smoothie journey, but all the good habits that add to your well-being.

- **Beyond Smoothies**

This tracker goes beyond the delicious green recipes. It's like your personal helper, helping you keep tabs on other healthy habits that add up to a better you. Exercise, hydration, or a good night's sleep – check, check, and check!

- **Checkboxes, Sliders, and Emojis**

Making tracking fun is the name of the game. Think of checks as little wins waiting to be marked. Sliders make it easy to measure progress. Emojis add a touch of fun – happy faces for finished jobs or thumbs up for hitting your goals. It's like changing tracking into a joyful and expressive experience.

- **Proud Moments in a Box**

Every checkbox is a happy moment recorded. It's like collecting small wins throughout the day. When you glance at your tracker, you see a visual reflection of your commitment to a better lifestyle.

• A Holistic Well-Being Tracker

This isn't just about tracking; it's about accepting overall well-being. Your habits, both big and small, add to the colorful picture of your health. It's like making a snapshot of your daily choices and their positive effect.

• Personalized and Adaptable

The Daily Habit Tracker is like an open friend. It reacts to your tastes. Checkboxes for ease, sliders for accuracy, and emojis for a bit of personality. It's like having a tool that fits perfectly into your lifestyle.

• Positive Reward

Checking off each habit becomes a moment of positive reward. It's like giving yourself a pat on the back for making good choices. The tracker changes into a visual sign of your commitment and progress.

- **A Daily Reflection**

Imagine using the tracker as a daily reflection tool. It's like taking a moment to appreciate the efforts you put into different parts of your well-being. Whether it's a happy face or a filled checkbox, each piece is a sign of your devotion.

So, think of your Daily Habit Tracker as more than just a list; it's your daily partner in building a healthy you. It makes tracking into a positive and interactive experience, pushing you to enjoy every step of your wellness path.

3. Mood & Energy Meter

Mood & Energy Meter is your personal compass, guiding you through the emotional landscape of your 30-day green smoothie adventure. It's like a mood diary with a twist − a tool to help you understand how your green habits influence not just your body but also your overall well-being.

- **Simple Scales and Smileys**

This is your emotional canvas. Picture simple scales or smiley faces representing your mood and energy levels. It's like painting a daily portrait of how you feel. The scales let you measure, and the smileys add a touch of positivity to your reflection.

- **Charting Your Emotional Well-Being**

The Mood & Energy Meter isn't just about tracking; it's about creating a visual representation of your emotional journey. It's like turning your emotions into a colorful graph, allowing you to see patterns and trends over time.

- **Understanding Impact**

Imagine each entry on the meter as a story. It's like creating a narrative of how your green habit impacts your mood and energy. Whether it's a boost in energy after a morning smoothie or a calming effect in the evening, your meter becomes a record of positive changes.

- **Reflective Moments**

Using the meter becomes a moment of reflection. It's like pausing to acknowledge how your choices influence your emotional well-being. Each entry is a reminder that your green smoothie adventure isn't just about physical health but also about feeling good inside.

- **Positive and Mindful Tracking**

This isn't about rating your mood; it's about expressing it. The meter transforms tracking into a positive and mindful experience. It's like giving yourself the space to explore and understand your emotional responses, fostering a deeper connection with your well-being.

- **Identifying Patterns**

As the days unfold on your Mood & Energy Meter, imagine noticing patterns. It's like discovering correlations between your green habits and how you feel. This awareness becomes a valuable tool, empowering you to make choices that positively impact your mood and energy.

- **Daily Well-Being Snapshot**

Think of the meter as a snapshot of your daily well-being. It's like capturing the essence of your emotions in a single glance. When you look back, you see not just the physical changes but also the emotional journey you've traveled.

So, your Mood & Energy Meter is more than a tracking tool; it's your emotional companion on this adventure. It adds a layer of mindfulness, helping you understand and appreciate the holistic impact of your green smoothie journey on your mood and energy.

4. Weekly Challenges

Consider the Weekly Challenges as exciting goals in your 30-day green smoothie journey. These tasks are meant to add a sprinkle of variety, keep things interesting, and provide you with chances to explore new parts of health. It's like having a weekly task that turns your trip into a dynamic and evolving experience.

- **Trying New Green Veggies**

Think of this task as a culinary adventure. It's like an offer to step out of your comfort zone and try a new green food in your smoothie. Whether it's kale, spinach, or something more exotic, each week becomes a chance to discover fresh tastes and nutritional benefits.

- **Incorporating Mindfulness Practices**

Imagine working awareness into your daily routine. This task is like a call to add mindfulness techniques alongside your green smoothie routine. It could be a few minutes of meditation, deep breathing movements, or simply enjoying your smoothie with full attention. It's a weekly lesson to feed not just your body but also your mind.

- **Sharing Smoothie Creations Online**

Picture this task as a virtual party. It's like pushing you to share your smoothie creations with the internet community. Whether through photos, recipes, or inspiring stories, this challenge turns your trip into a shared experience. It's a chance to meet, inspire, and be inspired by others on similar journeys.

• Adding a Dash of Creativity

Think of this challenge as an artistic project. It's like putting imagination into your smoothie-making process. Experiment with presentation, make bright layers, or design a themed smoothie. This task makes your daily routine into a canvas for self-expression and innovation.

• Bonus Nutritional Boost

Imagine going deeper into the world of eating. This challenge is like an extra quest to explore a special nutritional feature. It could involve adding a superfood like chia seeds, playing with plant-based proteins, or focusing on a particular vitamin-rich item. Each week becomes a chance to improve the nutritional profile of your smoothies.

• Weekly Reflections

Think of this task as a moment of thought. It's like making a weekly routine to think on your journey. Consider what worked well, any difficulties you faced, and the lessons learned. This reflective exercise adds a layer of awareness, making each week into a stepping stone for personal growth.

- **Celebrating Achievements**

Picture this challenge as a weekly party. It's like setting aside a moment to honor and celebrate your successes. Whether it's finishing a tough week or trying a new smoothie variation, this task turns your wins into joyful milestones.

So, your Weekly Challenges are more than just jobs; they're dynamic elements that bring variety, inspiration, and a sense of satisfaction to your green smoothie adventure. Each task becomes a stepping stone in your journey, making your 30 days into a series of interesting and rewarding experiences.

5. Bonus Boosters

Imagine Bonus Boosters as unexpected treats during your 30-day green smoothie experience. These are like small jewels placed throughout your trip, offering an added layer of motivation, inspiration, and wisdom. They're meant to make your experience richer and more pleasurable, converting your regular routine into a discovery-filled adventure.

- **Inspirational Quotes**

Think of this booster as a dose of inspiration. It's like discovering a piece of knowledge each day. Whether it's a phrase on resilience, health, or the thrill of accepting change, these bites become your daily upliftment, bringing optimism to your path.

- **Fun Facts About Superfoods**

Picture this booster as a mini-lesson in nutrition. It's like finding intriguing facts about the superfoods in your smoothies. From the benefits of kale to the antioxidants in berries, these morsels of wisdom make your daily routine not just enjoyable but also enlightening.

- **Healthy Recipe Tips**

Imagine this booster as a creative spark in your culinary quest. It's like receiving advice and ideas to boost your smoothie recipes. Whether it's a new mix, a presentation idea, or a taste match, these suggestions turn your everyday blending into a gourmet journey.

- **Daily Affirmations**

Think of this booster as positive reinforcement. It's like receiving affirmations that applaud your dedication. Whether it's appreciating your devotion or recognizing the great improvements you're making, these daily affirmations offer a source of support on your journey.

- **Wellness Challenges**

Picture this booster as an extra experience within your trip. It's like adding a mini-challenge to your routine. It may be a call to take an additional stroll, try a new kind of exercise, or practice thankfulness. These challenges invigorate your daily life with diversity and total well-being.

- **Mindful Moments**

Imagine this booster as a reminder to be present. It's like putting moments of awareness into your day. Whether it's a cue for deep breathing, a quick meditation suggestion, or a thoughtful smoothie-sipping activity, these moments bring serenity to your journey.

- **Recipe of the Day**

Think of this booster as a gastronomic surprise. It's like presenting a highlighted recipe to try. Whether it's a refreshing green smoothie variant, a nutrient-packed addition, or a themed creation, these ideas make your daily routine intriguing and delectable.

So, Bonus Boosters are more than simply additional nutrients; they're like hidden treasures that make your green smoothie trip not only healthy for your body but also enriching for your mind and spirit. Each booster provides a new flavor to your trip, making every day a discovery and celebration.

6. Achievement Stickers

Celebrate your milestones with playful stickers. Visualize Achievement Stickers as your customized badges of honor on this 30-day green juice journey.

These stickers are like bright rewards that celebrate your goals and successes, transforming your progress into a visually engaging and uplifting experience.

- **Completion of Key Weeks**

Imagine this sticker as a badge of resilience. It's like getting a golden star for finishing important milestones, such as the end of each week. Each sticker becomes a symbol of your loyalty and success, turning your calendar into a canvas of victories.

- **Conquering the Entire Challenge**

Think of this sticker as the big prize. It's like unlocking a special badge for successfully finishing the entire 30-day task. This sticker marks the end of your trip, a testament to your commitment to a healthier living.

- **Trying New Smoothie Variations**

Picture this sticker as a mark of creativity. It's like putting a sticker for discovering and playing with new smoothie variations. Whether it's a unique blend of ingredients or a creative presentation, each sticker becomes a colorful tribute to your cooking experiences.

- **Meeting Nutritional Goals**

Imagine this sticker as a healthy success. It's like getting a sticker for regularly meeting your daily nutritional goals. Whether it's hitting the recommended amount of vitamins or incorporating diverse superfoods, these stickers become a visual reflection of your commitment to well-rounded health.

- **Consistent Exercise Accomplishments**

Think of this sticker as a sign of energy. It's like getting a sticker for regularly integrating exercise into your habit. Whether it's a daily walk, a workout session, or yoga practice, these stickers become a lively reflection of your commitment to overall well-being.

- **Sharing Achievements Online**

Picture this tag as a digital applause. It's like getting a sticker for sharing your achievements with the internet community. Each shared success story, recipe, or picture becomes a virtual celebration, and the sticker is your badge of involvement in a supportive and inspiring community.

- **Mindful Eating Recognition**

Imagine this sticker as a moment of thought. It's like getting a sticker for adopting mindful eating habits. Whether it's enjoying each sip of your smoothie or being present during meals, these stickers become a memory of your mindfulness journey.

So, Achievement Stickers are more than just decorations; they're like joyful marks of your progress, changing your 30-day green smoothie trip into a visual party. Each sticker is a symbol of your successes, making your trip vibrant, engaging, and a source of continuous inspiration.

Your Smart Weight Loss Device: Your Personal Coach

Envision your Smart Weight Loss Device as a trusted personal coach accompanying you on your 30-day green smoothie adventure. This device is not just a scale; it's a sophisticated tool designed to provide personalized insights, support your weight loss goals, and enhance your overall well-being:

1. Choose Your Champion

Selecting your champion in the form of a Smart Weight Loss Device is a key choice, akin to choosing a trusted partner for your 30-day green smoothie path. This decision-making process includes a thoughtful review of your weight management goals and the specific data points that resonate with your tastes and needs.

- **Smart Scale**

__Functionality:__ A smart scale is more than just a standard scale. It offers advanced features such as measuring weight, body fat percentage, and sometimes additional measures like muscle mass and water weight.

Data Precision: It offers exact data, allowing you to track your weight loss journey with accuracy. Some smart scales can even connect to apps or devices to share your data effortlessly.

- **Fitness Tracker**

Comprehensive Monitoring: A fitness tracker goes beyond weight measurement, giving a wider spectrum of health data. It usually tracks your daily physical activity, heart rate, sleep patterns, and sometimes even stress levels.

Real-time Feedback: With real-time feedback on your daily actions, a fitness watch becomes an engaging Companion. It motivates you to stay active, meet step goals, and keep a holistic approach to health.

- **Body Composition Analyzer**

In-Depth Insights: This gadget goes beyond basic weight measurement. It offers detailed insights into your body makeup, including the amount of muscle, fat, water, and bone. This comprehensive view is important for those wanting a deeper understanding of their physical health.

Goal-specific Analysis: If your weight management goals require specific changes in body composition, a body composition analyzer becomes a smart choice. It helps direct your efforts toward reaching a desired balance.

- **Reflect on Goals**

Consider your main goals. If weight loss is the central goal, a smart scale might serve. If you aim for a holistic method covering various health factors, a fitness tracker or body composition analyzer could be more ideal.

- **Preferred Metrics**

Identify the exact data points that connect with your goals. Whether it's tracking steps, watching body fat percentage, or having a complete overview of body composition, choose the measures that match with your goals.

- **User-Friendly Interface**

Evaluate the user interface and compatibility of the device with your tracking system. A seamless connection between your chosen hero and the progress tracker ensures a unified and user-friendly experience.

In essence, picking your winner involves matching the features and capabilities of your Smart Weight Loss Device with your unique health journey. It becomes the guiding beacon, giving insights, encouragement, and a personalized path towards meeting your health goals during the 30-day green smoothie plan.

2. Sync & Track: Keeping Things Simple and Connected

Imagine Sync & Track as the magic that makes your Smart Weight Loss Device and progress tracker work together effortlessly during your 30-day green smoothie adventure.

- **Easy Connection**

Sync & Track is like a magical link that connects your Smart Weight Loss Device to your progress tracker. It's simple and works like a charm, making sure your data flows smoothly.

- **All-in-One Information**

Everything Together: This feature brings all your health info together in one place. Your weight, exercise, and other important details sync up, giving you a complete picture of how you're doing on your health journey.

- **Instant Updates**

Right Away: It's like getting instant updates. As you sync, you see how you're doing in real-time. No waiting around – just quick updates on your progress.

- **See Your Progress**

Picture This: Sync & Track helps you see your progress visually. Imagine graphs and charts that show how well you're doing. It's like having a map to guide you on your health adventure.

- **Easy Goal Setting**

Your Plan, Your Way: With Sync & Track,

setting and changing your goals is easy. It's like
being the boss of your health journey, adjusting
things as you go to make sure you're on the right
track.

In simple terms, Sync & Track is the cool feature
that makes sure your Smart Weight Loss Device
and progress tracker talk to each other nicely. It's
like having a helpful friend that keeps everything
simple and connected, so you can focus on enjoying
your green smoothie journey.

3. Visualize Progress

Imagine Visualize Progress as the tool that turns
your Smart Weight Loss Device data into a clear
picture of how you're doing on your 30-day green
smoothie trip.

1. See the Changes Like a Movie

Visualize Progress is like watching a movie of your
health journey. It takes the info from your Smart
Weight Loss Device and turns it into a story you can

see. You get a front-row seat to watch the changes happening over time.

2. Easy-to-Understand Graphics

Think of Visualize Progress as an artist making pictures. It uses easy-to-understand graphs and maps, not difficult numbers. It's like seeing your health journey as bright pictures that tell you how well you're doing.

• 3. Highlights of Success

Visualize Progress is like a spotlight on your successes. It shows the days you did really well – maybe you hit your exercise goal or stayed on track with your drinks. It's a way of enjoying your successes.

4. Identify Patterns

Connect the Dots: With Visualize Progress, you can connect the dots. It helps you see trends – maybe you feel better on days you have more green drinks. It's like having a spy tool that reveals what works best for you.

5. Adjust Your Course

Your Personal GPS: Think of Visualize Progress as your guidance system. If you see a dip in your progress, it's like a gentle warning to change your direction. It helps you stay on the right road towards your health goals.

In simple words, Visualize Progress is the cool tool that takes your health data and turns it into pictures. It's like having a visual guide that shows how awesome you're doing on your green smoothie trip, making it easy to understand and celebrate your successes along the way.

4. Goal Setting

Goal Setting is like making your own treasure map for the 30-day green smoothie journey. It's a way to decide where you want to go, set realistic goals, and keep yourself inspired on the path to a healthier lifestyle.

- **Choose Your Destination**

- Where You Want to Be:

Goal Setting is like picking a location. Maybe it's dropping weight, being more athletic, or having a daily green smoothie. It's about knowing what you want to achieve during your 30-day journey.

- **Break It Into Steps**

- Small, Achievable Goals: Think of Goal Setting as breaking your big goal into smaller steps. It's like setting milestones that are easy to reach. Each step is a win, making the whole journey feel less overwhelming.

- **Make It Your Own**

- Personalized Plans: Goal Setting is designed just for you. It's like having a plan that fits your lifestyle and health choices. Whether you're working on exercise, nutrition, or both, it's a plan built around what works best for you.

- **Stay Inspired**

- Your Own Motivator: With Goal Setting, it's

like being your own cheerleader. Achieving each milestone becomes a source of inspiration. It keeps you excited and committed to your journey, turning your goals into uplifting wins.

- **Adjust as You Go**

- *Flexible Route:* Think of Goal Setting as an open tool. If you need to change your goals – maybe adding more exercise or trying new drink recipes – it's easy to adjust. It's like having a plan that changes to your changing needs.

Goal Setting is your way of planning the journey. It's like making a plan that guides you towards success, one step at a time. It makes your 30-day green smoothie journey personal, doable, and truly yours.

5. Personalized Insights

Imagine Personalized Insights as your personal health detective during the 30-day green smoothie journey. It's like having a guide that uncovers unique information about your well-being.

- **Tailored Information**

- *Just for You:* Personalized Insights is like having a guidebook crafted specifically for your health journey. It provides information that suits your body and preferences. It's not one-size-fits-all – it's all about what works best for you.

- **Advanced Understanding**

- *Deeper Insights:* Think of Personalized Insights as a magnifying glass. It goes beyond the basics, providing detailed information about your sleep, stress levels, and overall activity. It's like having a sneak peek into different aspects of your well-being.

- **Optimize Your Habits**

- *Fine-tuning Strategies:* With Personalized Insights, it's like having a strategy session. It helps you understand how your habits, like daily smoothie intake or exercise, impact your overall health. It's a tool to fine-tune your routines for maximum well-being.

- **Adapt to Your Needs**

- *Flexible Recommendations:* Imagine Personalized Insights as a wise friend who understands your changing needs. It offers recommendations based on your evolving health journey. It's like having advice that adapts to what your body requires.

- **Holistic Wellness Support**
- *Comprehensive Guidance:* Personalized Insights is not just about one thing. It's like a holistic support system, offering guidance on various aspects of your well-being. It helps you see the bigger picture and make informed choices for a healthier you.

Personalized Insights is like having a health expert by your side. It tailors information, gives you a deeper understanding of your body, and offers guidance that adapts to your unique needs during your 30-day green smoothie adventure. It's your personalized health companion, making the journey more insightful and enjoyable.

Beyond the 30 Days

As you wrap up your 30-day green smoothie trip, it's important to think about the road ahead. Consider these steps to keep your improved health habits and continue thriving beyond the original 30 days:

- **Acknowledge Your Wins**

Take a moment to enjoy your achievements during the 30 days. Whether it's finishing the task or meeting personal goals, recognizing your efforts improves motivation for the next step.

- **Reflect on Learnings**

Reflect on what you've learned about your body, habits, and tastes. Identify good improvements and places for improvement. This self-awareness is important for long-term health.

- **Set Long-Term Goals**

Consider your health goals beyond the original 30 days. Set reasonable and sustainable long-term goals. This could include keeping a certain weight, continuing regular exercise, or constantly adding green smoothies into your diet.

• Integrate New Habits

Build on Progress: Identify the habits from the task that brought the most advantage. Integrate these into your daily practice. Whether it's regular exercise, careful eating, or specific diet choices, make them a lasting part of your lifestyle.

• Community Support

Stay Connected: If you participated with a group during the challenge, continue to stay connected. Share your triumphs, difficulties, and experiences. A supportive group offers ongoing drive and encouragement.

• Periodic Challenges

Keep it Fresh: Consider periodic challenges to keep energy and drive. These could be mini-challenges focused on specific parts of health. Keeping things fresh avoids monotony and fuels your passion.

- **Regular Check-Ins**

Assess Your Progress: Schedule regular check-ins with yourself. Assess your work, reassess goals, and make changes as needed. Regular reviews help you stay responsible and on track.

- **Expand Your Wellness Toolkit**

Explore More: Continue studying different parts of wellness. Whether it's trying new foods, adding diverse exercises, or exploring mindfulness practices, widening your tools keeps your health journey dynamic.

- **Mindful Choices**

Conscious Decisions: Practice attention in your daily choices. Be aware of what you eat, how you move, and your general well-being. Mindful choices add to ongoing health gains.

- **Enjoy the Journey**

Embrace the Process: Remember that the road to a healthier you is continuing. Embrace the process, and view each day as a chance to make good choices. Enjoying the trip makes the goal of wellness more fulfilling.

By adding these tactics, you extend the positive effect of your 30-day green smoothie challenge. The habits developed during this time become the basis for a sustainable and ongoing journey towards a healthier, more vibrant lifestyle.

Multiple Formats, One Goal: Flexibility for Your Health Journey

The idea of "Multiple Formats, One Goal" is all about offering flexibility for people participating in the 30-day green smoothie challenge. By offering various forms, we hope to cater to diverse tastes and technological comfort levels, ensuring that everyone can start on their health journey with ease.

1. Printable Worksheet - Tangible and Traditional

For those who prefer a hands-on method, we offer a printed worksheet. It's like having a tangible guide that you can touch, write on, and pin up for daily exposure. This classic style appeals to those who enjoy a real link to their health plan.

2. Interactive Online Tool - Tech-Savvy Experience

The interactive online tool is created for people comfortable with technology. It offers a dynamic digital experience, allowing users to track progress, set goals, and access information with just a few clicks. It's like having your health guide available at your hands.

3. Customizable App -On-the-Go Convenience

The customized app takes the digital experience a step further. It's created for those who prefer controlling their health journey on the go. Like having a personalized health assistant in your pocket, the app offers convenience and real-time recording.

By offering these different formats, our goal is to suit various tastes and lifestyles. Whether you prefer the physical feel of a worksheet, the interactive nature of an online tool, or the ease of a mobile app, the core remains the same, to help you towards a healthier, more vibrant you. It's about making the 30-day green smoothie challenge available to all, independent of your chosen format.

Remember:

This system is your empowering partner, not a strict rulebook:

- Adapt it to your needs, adjust goals as needed, and, most importantly, have fun charting your path to a greener, leaner, and healthier you!

So, grab your blender, pick your smart device, and unleash your inner green warrior! With your personalized Smart Tracking System as your guide, your 30-day journey promises to be delicious, rewarding, and empowering.

How The Healthy Smoothie Plan is Impacting Your Well-being

As you begin on your health journey, take time to consider how the plan is affecting your overall well-being. Consider the following principles to promote attentive contemplation:

1. Physical Sensations

Take note of how your body feels after implementing the healthy green smoothie plan into your daily routine. Take note of changes in energy levels, digestion, and other bodily feelings that may signal beneficial alterations.

2. Mental Clarity and Focus

Assess your mental condition throughout the day. Are you feeling more clear and focused? A nutrient-dense diet can improve both physical and cognitive function.

3. Emotional Well-being

Examine your emotions and moods. Do you feel more optimistic, motivated, or emotionally balanced? Green smoothies include nutrients that can help with emotional well-being.

4. Sleep Quality

Consider how the plan may affect your sleep patterns. Many variables, including nutrition, can influence the quality of your sleep. Consider any improvements or changes you see in your sleep.

5. Proper Hydration

Maintain proper hydration levels with smoothies and enough water intake. Hydration is critical to general health, impacting a variety of biological systems.

6. Physical Activity and Mobility

Consider how the strategy fits with your physical activity. Are you feeling more motivated to move your body? A well-nourished body is more likely to respond to exercise and daily activities.

7. Social Connection

Wellness is more than simply nutrition; it's also about relationships. Consider how the plan could be affecting your social relationships. Are you sharing recipes, experiences, or even smoothies with your friends and family?

8. Mindful Eating Habits

Consume green smoothies with mindfulness. Consider the sensations of taste, the sustenance each drink delivers, and how this attention affects your entire connection with food.

9. Stress Levels

Evaluate the influence on your stress level. Nutrient-dense diets can help with stress resiliency. Consider whether you feel more prepared to handle everyday challenges.

10. Personal Achievements

Celebrate important milestones in your path. Take a moment to ponder your achievements, even those that may seem small or minor. Recognize your commitment to your health and the great measures you have done.

Remember that wellbeing is a comprehensive term that includes physical, mental, and emotional components. Regular reflection on these aspects will help you recognize the good improvements and drive you to continue caring for your total well-being with the 30-Days Healthy Green Smoothie Program.

Conclusion

As we reach the final pages of the 30 Days Healthy Green Smoothie Plan, it's time to reflect on the journey we've taken together. This book has been your guide to a healthier lifestyle, and as we wrap it up, let's highlight the key lessons and celebrate the positive changes you've made.

1. The Journey Towards Health

Over the past 30 days, you embarked on a journey towards a healthier you. It wasn't about complicated diets or strict rules; it was about making small, manageable changes that contribute to your well-being.

2. The Power of Green Smoothies

The heart of this plan was the green smoothie – a simple concoction of fruits and leafy greens. These nutrient-packed drinks became your allies, providing essential vitamins and minerals that your body craves for energy and vitality.

3. Holistic Wellness Approach

This book encouraged a holistic approach to wellness. It wasn't just about what you ate; it was about moving your body, being mindful of your choices, and finding support in a community that shares similar goals.

4. Tracking Your Progress

The tracking system introduced in the book helped you monitor your progress. Whether through a simple calendar or a digital app, keeping tabs on your daily choices allowed you to see how far you've come and celebrate your victories.

5. Community Support

Connecting with others on a similar journey provided a sense of camaraderie. Sharing experiences, challenges, and triumphs created a supportive community. Together, you found strength in knowing that you're not alone in your pursuit of a healthier life.

6. Reflective Journaling

Taking a few minutes each day to jot down your thoughts and reflections in the provided journal allowed you to build a deeper connection with your wellness journey. It became a personal space to acknowledge challenges, celebrate successes, and learn more about yourself.

7. Flexibility in Choices

This plan emphasized flexibility. It wasn't about rigid rules but about finding what works for you. Whether you preferred a printable worksheet or a mobile app, the goal was to make the journey adaptable to your lifestyle.

8. Long-Term Wellness

As we conclude this book, it's important to recognize that the 30-day plan isn't just a short-term fix. The habits you've cultivated are seeds for long-term wellness. The goal is for these changes to become a natural part of your daily life, contributing to sustained health.

9. Your Continued Journey

The book is closing, but your wellness journey continues. It's about taking the lessons learned – the power of green smoothies, the importance of movement, mindful choices, and community support and incorporating them into your ongoing lifestyle.

10. Cheers to Your Health

Here's to you and your commitment to a healthier tomorrow! The book may be ending, but the story of your well-being is just beginning. Continue making choices that nourish your body, mind, and spirit. Cheers to a healthier, more vibrant you!

In wrapping up the 30 Days Healthy Green Smoothie Plan, remember that the journey to better health is ongoing. Let the lessons learned guide you, and may each day bring you closer to a life filled with vitality and well-being.